Bates Method Nuggets

Bates Method Nuggets

The Fundamentals of
Natural Vision Improvement
by William H. Bates, M.D.

Compiled by Esther Joy van der Werf

Bates Method Nuggets
ISBN: 978-1-935894-13-1

Published by Visions of Joy
10239 Ojai Santa Paula Rd
Ojai, CA 93023, USA
www.visionsofjoy.org

Cover Design by Leideke Steur & Tatiana Swope

Foreword

Ojai, California, 7 July 2010

Dear Reader,

On the following pages you will find the 'golden nuggets' of the Bates Method of natural eyesight improvement. These are true gems, in their original form, the way Dr. William H. Bates published them in his monthly *Better Eyesight* magazines in the 1920s.

Out of the 132 magazines containing hundreds of pages, Dr. Bates suggested that each magazine's 'page 2' should be kept for reference and frequent review.

This book brings these 'page 2' gems together, sorted by subject, and presents them to you in an order that will help you gain a good overall understanding of the Bates Method. This understanding comes step by step, page by page, in an easy and logical flow from one subject to the next.

When you read this book once, you'll deepen your understanding of your own vision and how you can improve it yourself. When re-read from time to time, it will help you continue to make progress toward effortless clear vision and it will help you keep your good eyesight.

I wish you all the best on your path to clarity!

Love & Light,
Esther

Esther Joy van der Werf
www.VisionsOfJoy.org
Natural Eyesight Improvement

Better Eyesight
A monthly magazine devoted to the prevention
and cure of imperfect sight without glasses.

"Page Two"

On page two of this magazine are printed each month specific directions for improving the sight in various ways. Too many subscribers read the magazine once and then mislay it. We feel that at least page two should be kept for reference.

When the eyes are neglected the vision may fail. It is so easy to forget how to palm successfully. The long swing always helps but it has to be done right. One may under adverse conditions suffer a tension so great that the ability to remember or imagine perfectly is modified or lost and relaxation is not obtained. The long swing is always available and always brings sufficient relief to practice the short swing, central fixation, the perfect memory and imagination with perfect relief.

Be sure and review page two frequently; not only for your special benefit but also for the benefit of individuals you desire to help!

Persons with imperfect sight often have difficulty in obtaining relaxation by the various methods described in the book and in this magazine. It should be emphasized that persons with good vision are better able to help others than people who have imperfect sight or wear glasses. If you are trying to cure yourself avoid people who wear glasses or do not see well. Those individuals are always under a strain and the strain is manifested in their face, in their voices, in their walk, the way they sit, in short in everything that they do.

Strain is contagious. Teachers in Public Schools who wear glasses are a menace to their pupils' sight. Parents who wear glasses or who have imperfect sight lower the vision of their children. It is always well when treating children or adults to keep them away from people with imperfect sight.

William H. Bates, M.D., July 1922

Table of Contents

1. GLASSES

No Glasses For Quick Results

The first and best thing that all patients should do after their first treatment, or before, is to discard their glasses. It is not always an easy thing to do but it is best for the patient and for the teacher. It is true that at one time I did not encourage patients to learn the treatment unless they discarded their glasses permanently. But since I have studied more about my method and have encouraged some of my clinic patients to wear their glasses at times while under treatment, I find that some of them obtained a cure but it required double the amount of time that was required to cure those who discarded their glasses permanently. During the treatment when the glasses are worn temporarily, even for a short time, the vision sometimes becomes worse and in most cases a relapse is produced. It is much more difficult to regain the lost ground than ever before, and sometimes causes much discomfort.

Glasses for the correction of myopia do not fit the eyes all the time. To obtain good vision with glasses an effort is required to make the eyes change their focus to have the same error of refraction as the glasses correct. When the vision is benefited most perfectly by glasses it is necessary for the eyes to change frequently. To learn the amount of myopia in the eyes by trying different glasses to find the glass which continuously improves the vision best is usually difficult because the amount of the myopia changes so frequently. To change the amount of myopia requires an effort. Some people complain that no glasses fit their eyes permanently. These cases are benefited by discarding their glasses for a longer or a shorter period while being treated. Patients who require good sight to earn a living and find it difficult to discard their glasses while under treatment, have been able to make slow or rapid progress in the cure of their imperfect sight by wearing their glasses only when it was absolutely necessary.

GLASSES

Discard Glasses

Easy to say, something else to do. But it is a fact that no one can be cured without glasses and wear glasses at the same time.

This is a fact that one should keep in mind. It may help to give one backbone sufficient to do the right thing. I know how difficult it is from personal experience. I suppose I have as much originality, if not more, than the average person. It required a year before I was convinced that my eyes could not be cured unless I stopped wearing glasses. I could not wear them even for emergencies without suffering a relapse.

Patients who are really anxious to be cured can discard glasses and obtain benefit almost from the start. Wearing of glasses becomes a fixed habit. The idea of going without them is a shock. The honest determination to do all that is possible to be done for a cure, makes it easy or easier to discard glasses at once. Patients tell me that after they have discarded their glasses for a few days they do not feel as uncomfortable as they expected.
Do not use opera glasses. Do not use a magnifying glass for any purpose.

It is very natural that one should hesitate to discard glasses after he has worn them for many years and obtained what seems considerable benefit. It may help to read what I have published about glasses. Most of the discomforts of the eyes are largely functional or nervous and not due to any real or organic trouble with the eyes. All the symptoms of discomfort are accompanied by a strain which produces a wrong focus of the eyes called myopia, hypermetropia, astigmatism or presbyopia. Glasses may correct the wrong focus produced by the strain, but they do not always, because the eyes are not always strained to fit glasses accurately. While wearing glasses in order to see, one has to strain or, by an effort, squeeze the eye ball out of shape and it is impossible therefore, to obtain relaxation and see with glasses.

If one can understand what I have just stated one can realize the necessity of discarding glasses in order to obtain a cure. I feel that the facts should be emphasized and the patient made to understand the necessity of discarding glasses. This makes it easier for the patient to do without glasses.

Do not argue with yourself about the matter. When you go to a doctor you expect to take his medicine even though you may not know what it is or how it is going to act. When patients come to me for relief I say, "Discard your glasses and you can be cured." If they are wise they do as I say without any talk.

Demonstrate

That glasses lower the vision.

Stand fifteen feet from the Snellen test card* and test the vision of each eye without glasses. Then test the vision of each eye with glasses on, after having worn them for half an hour or longer. Remove the glasses; test the vision again and compare the results. Note that the vision without glasses becomes better, the longer the glasses are left off.

Test the eyes of a person who is very nearsighted. Remove the glasses and test the sight of each eye at five feet, nearer or farther, until the distance is found at which the vision is best without glasses. Now test the vision for five minutes at this distance, which is the optimum distance, or the distance at which the vision is best. For example, nearsighted people see best when the print is held a foot or nearer to the eyes. If the eyes see best at six inches, the optimum distance is six inches; but if the distance at which the eyes see best is thirty to forty inches, the optimum distance is then thirty or forty inches.

In nearsightedness, glasses always lower the vision at the optimum distance. The same is true in farsightedness or astigmatism. For example, a nearsighted person may have an optimum distance of six inches. If glasses are worn, the vision is never as good at six inches as it is without them. This demonstrates that glasses lower the vision at six inches, or the optimum distance in this case. In farsightedness without glasses, the optimum distance, at which objects are seen best, may be ten feet or further. If glasses are worn and the sight is improved at a nearer point, the vision without glasses at the optimum distance becomes worse.

* The Snellen Test Card is the typical eye-chart used by eye doctors.

GLASSES

Curable Cases

Patients wearing glasses for the relief of imperfect sight may expect better vision after they are cured than they ever had before with glasses. Adults who have good distant vision but require glasses after middle life, for reading, are also curable without glasses. Such patients, although they may read very well with glasses, complain that, as a rule, they must hold the page at one distance in order to read with the best vision. This reading distance is usually about twelve inches.

Some cases require one pair of glasses for reading books or newspapers, but cannot see clearly at a greater distance without another pair of glasses. Musicians especially find that glasses that give them good vision for reading books are useless to them for reading music or for playing the piano. To see closer than twelve inches may require still another pair of glasses. To see more distant objects may require still another pair. Some of my patients have shown me numerous pairs of glasses, each one adapted for certain specific distances. It is a great relief to such cases to be cured, because then they are able, not only to see perfectly at the distance without glasses, but they can read the fine print as well at six inches as they can further off. The eye with normal sight is able to change its focus at will for all distances without any discomfort whatever.

Patients with cataract, glaucoma and other diseases of the eyes may not be able to see even with glasses. When they are cured by my methods they become able to see normally in all kinds of light, in a bright light or in a dim light. Pain, fatigue and other discomforts of the eyes are all relieved.

2. REST

Rest

All methods of curing errors of refraction are simply different ways of obtaining rest.

Different persons do this in different ways. Some patients are able to rest their eyes simply by closing them, and complete cures have been obtained by this means, the closing of the eyes for a longer or shorter period being alternated with looking at the test card for a moment. In other cases patients have strained more when their eyes were shut than when they were open.

Some can rest their eyes when all light is excluded from them by covering with the palms of the hands; others cannot, and have to be helped by other means before they can palm. Some become able at once to remember or imagine that the letters they wish to see are perfectly black, and with the accompanying relaxation their vision immediately becomes normal. Others become able to do this only after a considerable time.

Shifting is a very simple method of relieving strain, and most patients soon become able to shift from one letter to another, or from one side of a letter to another in such a way that these forms seem to move in a direction opposite to the movement of the eye. A few are unable to do this, but can do it with a mental picture of a letter, after which they become able to do it visually.

Patients who do not succeed with any particular method of obtaining rest for their eyes should abandon it and try something else. The cause of the failure is strain, and it does no good to go on straining.

The Palming Cure

One of the most efficacious methods of relieving eyestrain, and hence of improving the sight, is palming. By this is meant the covering of the closed eyes with the palms of the hands in such a way as to exclude all the light, while avoiding pressure upon the eyeballs. In this way most patients are able to secure some degree of relaxation in a few minutes, and when they open their eyes find their vision temporarily improved.

When relaxation is complete the patient sees, when palming, a black so deep that it is impossible to remember or imagine anything blacker, and such relaxation is always followed by a complete and permanent cure of all errors of refraction (nearsight, farsight, astigmatism and even old sight), as well as by the relief or cure of many other abnormal conditions. In rare cases patients become able to see a perfect black very quickly, even in five, ten or fifteen minutes; but usually this cannot be done without considerable practice, and some never become able to do it until they have been cured by other means. When the patient becomes able after a few trials to see an approximate black, it is worth while to continue with the method; otherwise something else should be tried.

Most patients are helped by the memory of some color, preferably black, and as it is impossible to remember an unchanging object for more than a few seconds, they usually find it necessary to shift consciously from one mental picture to another, or from one part of such a picture to another. In some cases, however, the shifting may be done unconsciously, and the black object may appear to be remembered all alike continuously.

Demonstrate

1. That palming improves the sight.

When both eyes are closed and covered with one or both hands in such a way as to exclude all light, one does not see red, blue, green or any other color. In short, when the palming is successful one does not see anything but black, and when the eyes are opened, the vision is always improved.

2. That an imperfect memory prevents perfect palming and the vision is lowered.

Remember a letter "O" imperfectly, a letter "O" which has no white center and is covered by a gray cloud. It takes time; the effort is considerable and in spite of all that is done, the memory of the imperfect "O" is lost or forgotten for a time. The whole field is a shade of gray or of some other color, and when the hands are removed from the eyes, the vision is lowered.

3. That when a perfect letter "O" is remembered, palming is practiced properly, continuously and easily and the sight is always benefited.

4. That to fail to improve the sight by palming, or to palm imperfectly is difficult. To fail, requires a stare or a strain and is not easy. When an effort is made the eyes and mind are staring, straining, trying to see. When no effort is made, the palming becomes successful and the vision is benefited. Successful palming is not accomplished by doing things. Palming becomes successful by the things that are not done.

5. That the longer you palm, the greater the benefit to your vision. Palm first for two minutes, then four minutes, six, etc., until you have palmed for fifteen. Notice the improvement gained in 15 minutes has been greater than that in four minutes.

The Flashing Cure

Do you read imperfectly? Can you observe then that when you look at the first word, or the first letter, of a sentence you do not see best where you are looking; that you see other words, or other letters, just as well as or better than the ones you are looking at? Do you observe also that the harder you try to see the worse you see?

Now close your eyes and rest them, remembering some color, like black or white, that you can remember perfectly. Keep them closed until they feel rested, or until the feeling of strain has been completely relieved. Now open them and look at the first word or letter of a sentence for a fraction of a second. If you have been able to relax, partially or completely, you will have a flash of improved or clear vision, and the area seen best will be smaller.

After opening the eyes for this fraction of a second, close them again quickly, still remembering the color, and keep them closed until they again feel rested. Then again open them for a fraction of a second. Continue this alternate resting of the eyes and flashing of the letters for a time, and you may soon find that you can keep your eyes open longer than a fraction of a second without losing the improved vision.

If your trouble is with distant instead of near vision, use the same method with distant letters.

In this way you can demonstrate for yourself the fundamental principles of the cure of imperfect sight by treatment without glasses.

If you fail, ask someone with perfect sight to help you.

Alternate

It has always been demonstrated that the continuous memory, imagination, or vision of one thing for any length of time is impossible. To see one letter of the Snellen test card continuously, it is necessary to shift from one part of the letter to another. By alternately moving the eyes from one side of the letter to the other, it is possible to imagine the letter to be moving in the opposite direction to the movement of the eyes. This movement of the letter is called a swing. When it is slow, easy, short, about one-quarter of an inch or less, maximum vision is obtained which continues as long as the swing continues.

As long as we are awake, we are thinking, remembering, or imagining mental pictures, and are comfortable. To go around blind requires a distinct effort which is a strain on all the nerves and is always uncomfortable. The normal mind alternates its attention from one mental picture to another, which is a relaxation or rest. The memory, or imagination, is best when one thing is imagined better than all other things, Central Fixation, but constant shifting is necessary to maintain Central Fixation.

One of the best methods to improve the vision is to regard a letter of the Snellen test card with the eyes open, then close the eyes and remember or imagine the letter better for about ten seconds, open the eyes and regard the letter while testing the imagination of the letter for a moment. By alternately regarding the letter with the eyes open and closed, the imagination of the letter improves in flashes. By continuing to alternate the flashes improve and last longer until the vision becomes continuously improved.

3. BLINKING

Blinking

The normal eye when it has normal sight rests very frequently by closing the eyes for longer or shorter periods, and when practiced quickly it is called BLINKING. When the normal eye has normal sight and refrains from blinking for some seconds or part of a minute, the vision always becomes imperfect. You can demonstrate that normal vision at the near point or at the distance is impossible without frequent blinking. Most people blink so easily and for such a short period of time that things are seen continuously while the blinking is done unconsciously. In some cases one may blink five times or more in one second. The frequency of blinking depends on a number of factors.

The normal eye blinks more frequently or more continuously under adverse conditions as when the illumination is diminished, the distance is increased or the print read is too pale or otherwise imperfect. The distraction of conversation, noise, reflections of light, objects so arranged as to be difficult to see, all increase the frequency of blinking of the normal eye with normal sight. If the frequency of blinking is diminished under adverse conditions or from any cause the vision soon becomes imperfect.

The imperfect eye or the eye with imperfect sight blinks less frequently than the normal eye. Staring stops the blinking. The universal optical swing, the long or short swing when modified or stopped are always accompanied by less frequent blinking.

Blink in the early morning.
Blink when the sun sets at night;
Blink when the sun is dawning,
But be sure you do it right.

Blinking

Blinking is one of the best methods that may be employed to obtain relaxation or rest. When rest is obtained by blinking, the vision is improved, not only for one letter or part of one letter, but for all the letters of a page, which may be seen some parts best, other parts not so well. This is called central fixation and one cannot see anything clearly without it. In order to maintain central fixation, there should be continuous opening and closing of the eyes by blinking which makes it easier for the vision to improve. When the eye discontinues to blink, it usually stares, strains, and tries to see. Blinking is beneficial only when practiced in the right way.

What is the right way? The question may be answered almost as briefly as it is asked. Blinking when done properly is slow, short, and easy. One may open and close the eyes an innumerable number of times in one second, and do so unconsciously.

Lord Macaulay was able to read a page of print in one second, and blinked for every letter. In order to read perfectly, he had to see each side of every letter by central fixation. We know that he acquired or had a perfect memory, because it was only with a perfect memory that he could recite the pages of any book which he had read many years before.

A casual observer would not be able to determine the number of times Lord Macaulay blinked, as it was done so quickly and easily, without any effort on his part. While most of us will not be able to blink without effort as frequently as Lord Macaulay did, it is well to practice his methods as well as we can. Those with imperfect sight who do not blink sufficiently should watch someone with normal eyes blink unconsciously and then imitate him.

4. EYESTRAIN

Stop Staring

It can be demonstrated by tests with the retinoscope that all persons with imperfect sight stare, strain, or try to see. To demonstrate this fact: Look intently at one part of a large or small letter at the distance or nearpoint. In a few seconds, usually, fatigue and discomfort will be produced, and the letter will blur or disappear. If the effort is continued long enough, pain may be produced.

To break the habit of staring:

(1) Shift consciously from one part to another of all objects regarded, and imagine that these objects move in a direction contrary to the movement of the eye. Do this with letters on the test card, with letters of fine print, if they can be seen, and with other objects.

(2) Close the eyes frequently for a moment or longer. When the strain is considerable, keep the eyes closed for several minutes and open them for a fraction of a second—flashing. When the stare is sufficient to keep the vision down to 2/200 or less, palm for a longer or shorter time; then look at the card for a moment. Later mere closing of the eyes may afford sufficient rest.

(3) Imagine that the white openings and margins of letters are whiter than the rest of the background. Do this with eyes closed and open alternately. It is an interesting fact that this practice prevents staring and improves the vision rapidly.

Demonstrate

That it requires an effort or a strain to produce imperfect sight.

Look at the notch at the top of the big "C" of the Snellen test card at fifteen feet. Keep your eyes fixed on the notch. Make an effort to see it and increase that effort as much as you possibly can. Notice that it is difficult to keep your eyes and mind fixed on that one point. Notice also that it is tiresome and makes your eyes pain. If you keep it up long enough, your head begins to ache and all the nerves of your body are strained.

If you look at some of the letters on the lower lines which are much smaller than the big "C", they may appear so blurred that you are not able to distinguish them. Trying to see these small letters blurs them still more.

Now hold the test card in your hand about one foot from your eyes. The big "C" is seen plainly and without any effort. Try to see the top and the bottom of the big "C" perfectly black at the same time. Notice that the "C" becomes blurred and the strain which blurs it also gives much discomfort.

From this evidence, we can conclude that perfect sight comes easily, without any effort or strain, while, imperfect sight is always produced by a strain or an effort to see.

Watch Your Step

When you know what is the matter with you it is possible for you to correct it and bring about a cure. If you do not know what is wrong with you the cure of your imperfect sight is delayed. Some persons have been cured quickly when they were able to demonstrate that to see imperfectly required a tremendous effort, an effort which was very difficult. Some persons are cured in one visit and they readily demonstrate that imperfect sight or failure to see is difficult. Others require weeks and months to demonstrate the facts. Perfect sight is quick, comes easy and without any effort whatever. Imperfect sight is slow, difficult. One cannot consciously make the sight worse as readily as it can be done unconsciously. There is no danger in demonstrating the facts.

Look at a small letter on the Snellen test card which can be seen clearly at ten or twenty feet, a letter O for example. When the letter is seen quite perfectly it is usually seen without any apparent effort. However, by looking intently, staring at it and making an effort to improve it the letter blurs. It can always be demonstrated that the effort to see very soon blurs the letter. Now close the eyes and rest them for a part of a minute or longer and then glance at the letter again. It will usually be as clear as it was before. Again by straining, making an effort, the letter becomes blurred. One can readily demonstrate that to make the sight worse requires an effort, a strain.

Many obstinate cases have obtained a permanent cure only after learning how to make the sight worse consciously. In my book are published Seven Truths of Normal Sight.* Prove the facts by demonstrating that the sight becomes imperfect when one or all of them is made imperfect by a strain.

* The book referred to is *Perfect Sight Without Glasses*, available from www.visionsofjoy.org. For the Seven Truths of Normal Sight see page 32 in this *Bates Method Nuggets* book.

Eyestrain

The eyes of all people with imperfect sight are under a strain. This is a truth. Most people believe that during sleep the eyes are at rest and that it is impossible to strain the eyes while sound asleep. This, however, is not true. Persons who have good sight in the daytime under favorable conditions may strain their eyes during sleep.

Many people awake in the morning suffering pain in the eyes or head. Often the eyes are very much fatigued and have a feeling of discomfort. There may be also a feeling of nervous tension from the eyestrain, or there may be a feeling as of sand in the eyes. At times all parts of the eye may be suffering from inflammation. The vision is sometimes lowered for several hours whereupon it begins to improve until it becomes as good as it was before the person retired the night before. Many people become alarmed and seek the services of some eye doctor. Usually the doctor or doctors consulted prescribe glasses which very rarely give more than imperfect or temporary relief.

There are various methods of correcting eyestrain occurring during sleep. Palming is very helpful even when practiced for a short time. A half an hour is often sufficient to relieve most if not all of the symptoms. In some cases the long swing, practiced before retiring, is sufficient to bring about temporary or permanent benefit. Blinking and shifting are also helpful. Good results have been obtained by practicing a perfect memory or imagination of one small letter of the Snellen test card alternately with the eyes open and closed. A number of patients were benefited and usually cured by remembering pleasant things perfectly.

Eyestrain During Sleep

Many people complain that when they first wake up in the morning, they are tired, that they have headaches, and that their sight is very imperfect. Later on in the day their eyes feel better, and the vision may become normal.

I have examined with the Ophthalmoscope the eyes of many people during sleep and found much to my surprise, that most people strain much more in their sleep than they ever do when they are awake. Of course, people when unconscious of their acts during sleep, are not aware of this eyestrain.

The prevention of eyestrain during sleep is usually a very difficult matter. Some cases are benefited just before retiring by palming for one-half hour or longer, or until they go to sleep while palming. Others by practicing the long swing for fifteen minutes, have found that the eyestrain becomes less. In some serious cases with imperfect sight, when the eyestrain is not prevented by palming or the swing, they are often materially benefited by shortening their hours of sleep with the help of an alarm clock. One patient had the alarm set for 3 am. He would then get out of bed and practice the long swing, alternating with palming for an hour or longer with the result that he slept the rest of the night very comfortably, and awoke the next morning with little or no evidence of eyestrain during sleep.

Some people have told me that they have lessened their eyestrain during sleep materially, by moderate muscular exercises for one-half hour or longer. They find that they obtain the best results when the exercise is continued sufficiently long to produce muscular fatigue.

Make Your Sight Worse

Strange as it may seem there is no better way of improving the sight than by making it worse. To see things worse when one is already seeing them badly requires mental control of a degree greater than that required to improve the sight. The importance of these facts is very great. When patients become able to lower their vision by conscious staring, they become better able to avoid unconscious staring. When they demonstrate by increasing their eccentric fixation that trying to see objects not regarded lowers the vision, they may stop trying to do the same thing unconsciously.

What is true of the sight is also true of the imagination and memory. If one's memory and imagination are imperfect, they can be improved by consciously making them worse than they are. Persons with imperfect sight never remember or imagine the letters on the test card as perfectly black and distinct, but to imagine them as grey and cloudy is very difficult, or even impossible, and when a patient has done it, or tried to do it, he may become able to avoid the unconscious strain which has prevented him from forming mental pictures as black and distinct as the reality.

To make imperfect sight worse is always more difficult than to lower normal vision. In other words, to make a letter which already appears grey and indistinct noticeably more cloudy is harder than to blur a letter seen distinctly. To make an imperfect mental picture worse is harder than to blur a perfect one. Both practices require much effort, much hard disagreeable work; but they always, when successful, improve the memory, imagination and vision.

Go To The Movies

Cinematograph pictures are commonly supposed to be very injurious to the eyes, and it is a fact that they often cause much discomfort and lowering of vision. They can, however, be made a means of improving the sight. When they hurt the eyes it is because the subject strains to see them. If this tendency to strain can be overcome, the vision is always improved, and, if the practice of viewing the pictures is continued long enough, nearsight, astigmatism and other troubles are cured.

If your sight is imperfect, therefore, you will find it an advantage to go to the movies frequently and learn to look at the pictures without strain. If they hurt your eyes, look away to the dark for a while, then look at a corner of the picture; look away again, and then look a little nearer to the center; and so on. In this way you may soon become able to look directly at the picture without discomfort. If this does not help, try palming for five minutes or longer. Dodge the pain, in short, and prevent the eyestrain by constant shifting, or by palming.

If you become able to look at the movies without discomfort, nothing else will bother you.

5. EYE-CHARTS

Suggestions

It is recommended by the editor of this magazine that every family should obtain a Snellen test card and place it on the wall of some room where it can be seen and read every day by all the members of the family. Not only does the daily reading of the card help the sight of children, but it is a benefit to the eyes of adults as well.

It is a well known fact that when most people arrive at the age of forty or fifty years, they find that their vision for reading or sewing is lowered. These people believe that they must put on glasses to prevent eyestrain, cataract, glaucoma, etcetera. Daily practice with the Snellen test card, together with the reading of fine print close to the eyes will overcome their difficulty.

Reading fine print close to the eyes, contrary to the belief of many ophthalmologists, is a benefit to the eyes of both children and adults.

It has been repeatedly demonstrated, however, that fine print cannot be read clearly or easily when an effort is made. When the eyes look directly at the letters, an effort is required, while looking at the white spaces between the lines is a rest, and by practice in this way, one can become able to see the letters clearly, without looking directly at them. When a patient looks at the white spaces between the lines of ordinary book type, he can read for hours and no fatigue, pain or discomfort is felt. When discomfort and pain in the eyes is felt while reading, it is because the patient is looking directly at the letters.

EYE-CHARTS

The Snellen Test Card

The Snellen Test Card is used for testing the eyesight. It is usually placed about 20 feet away from the patient. He covers each eye alternately, and reads the card as well as he can. Each line of letters is numbered with a figure which indicates the distance that it should be read with the normal eye.

When the vision is recorded it is written in the form of a fraction. The numerator being the distance of the patient from the card, and the denominator denoting the line read. For example:—If a patient at 10 feet can only read the line marked 100 the vision is written 10/100 or 1/10. If the patient at 20 feet can read the line marked 10 the vision is recorded as 20/10 which means that the sight is double that of the average eye.

Reading the Snellen Test Card daily helps the sight. Children in a public school with normal eyes under 12 years of age, who have never worn glasses were improved immediately by practicing with the Snellen Test Card. Children with imperfect sight also improved, and with the help of someone with perfect sight in time the vision becomes normal without glasses.

School children oftentimes are very much interested in their eyesight and what can be accomplished with the help of the Snellen Test Card. They have contests among themselves to see who can read the card best in a bright light, or on a rainy day when the light is dim. Many of them find out for themselves that straining makes the sight worse, while palming and swinging improve their vision. Many of them become able to use the Snellen Test Card in such a way as to relieve or prevent nervousness and headaches. Many boards of education hesitate to be responsible for any benefit that may be derived from the Snellen cards in the schools.

Distance Of The Snellen Test Card

The distance of the Snellen Test Card from the patient is a matter of considerable importance. Some patients improve more rapidly when the card is placed fifteen or twenty feet away while others fail to get any benefit with the card at this distance.

In some cases the best results are obtained when the card is as close as one foot. I recall a patient with very poor sight who made no progress whatever, when the card was placed at ten feet or further, but became able to improve the vision very materially with the card at about six inches. After the vision was improved at six inches the patient became able to improve the card at a greater distance until normal sight was obtained at twenty feet. Some cases with poor vision may not improve when the card is placed at ten feet or further, or at one foot or less but do much better when the card is placed at a middle distance, at about eight or ten feet. Other individuals may not improve their vision at all at ten feet, but are able to improve their sight at twenty feet or at one foot.

I recall one patient with 20 diopters of myopia whose vision at ten feet was peculiar. The letters at twenty feet and at one foot were apparently all the same normal size, but at ten feet they appeared to be one-fifth of the normal size. Practicing with the card at twenty feet or at one foot helped him greatly, more than practicing with the card at about ten feet. While some patients are benefited by practicing with the card daily always at the same distance, there are others who seem to be benefited when the distance of the card from the patient is changed daily.

How To Use The Snellen Test Card

for the Prevention and Cure of Imperfect Sight in Children

The Snellen Test Card is placed permanently upon the wall of the classroom, and every day the children silently read the smallest letters they can see from their seats with each eye separately, the other being covered with the palm of the hand in such a way as to avoid pressure on the eyeball. This takes no appreciable amount of time, and is sufficient to improve the sight of all children in one week and to cure all errors of refraction after some months, a year, or longer.

Children with markedly defective vision should be encouraged to read the card more frequently.

Records may be kept as follows:

John Smith, 10, Sept. 15, 1918.

R. V. (vision of the right eye) 20/40.
L. V. (vision of the left eye) 20/20.

John Smith, 11, Jan. 1, 1919.

R. V. 20/30.
L. V. 20/15.

The numerator of the fraction indicates the distance of the test card from the pupil; the denominator denotes the line read, as designated by the figures printed above the middle of each line of the Snellen Test Card.

A certain amount of supervision is absolutely necessary. At least once a year some one who understands the method should visit each classroom for the purpose of answering questions, encouraging the teachers to continue the use of the method, and making a report to the proper authorities.

It is not necessary that either the inspector, the teachers, or the children, should understand anything about the physiology of the eye.

Comparisons

In practicing with the Snellen test card, when the vision is imperfect, the blackness of the letters is modified and the white spaces inside the letters are also modified. By comparing the blackness of the large letters with the blackness of the smaller ones it can be demonstrated that the larger letters are imperfectly seen.

When one notes the whiteness in the center of a large letter, seen indistinctly, it is usually possible to compare the whiteness seen with the remembered whiteness of something else. By alternately comparing the whiteness in the center of a letter with the memory of a better white, as the snow on the top of a mountain, the whiteness of the letter usually improves. In the same way, comparing the shade of black of a letter with the memory of a darker shade of black of some other object may be also a benefit to the black.

Most persons with myopia are able to read fine print at a near point quite perfectly. They see the blackness and whiteness of the letters much better than they are able to see the blackness of the larger letters on the Snellen test card at 15 or 20 feet. Alternately reading the fine print and regarding the Snellen test card, comparing the black and white of the small letters with the black and white of the large letters, is often times very beneficial. Some cases of myopia have been cured very promptly by this method.

All persons with imperfect sight for reading are benefited by comparing the whiteness of the spaces between the lines with the memory of objects which are whiter. Many persons can remember white snow with the eyes closed whiter than the spaces between the lines. By alternately closing the eyes for a minute or longer, remembering white snow, white starch, white paint, a white cloud in the sky with the sun shining on it, and flashing the white spaces without trying to read, many persons have materially improved their sight and been cured.

Halos

When the eye with normal sight looks at the large letters on the Snellen test card, at any distance, from twenty feet to six inches or less, it sees, at the inner and outer edges and in the openings of the round letters, a white more intense than the margin of the card.

Similarly, when such an eye reads fine print, the spaces between the lines and the letters and the openings of the letters appear whiter than the margin of the page, while streaks of an even more intense white may be seen along the edges of the lines of letters. These "halos" are sometimes seen so vividly that in order to convince people that they are illusions it is often necessary to cover the letters, when they at once disappear.

Patients with imperfect sight also see the halos, though less perfectly, and when they understand that they are imagined, they often become able to imagine them where they had not been seen before, or to increase their vividness, in which case the sight always improves. This can be done by imagining the appearances first with the eyes closed; and then looking at the card, or at fine print, and imagining them there.

By alternating these two acts of imagination the sight is often improved rapidly. It is best to begin the practice at the point at which the halos are seen, or can be imagined best. Nearsighted patients are usually able to see them at the near-point, sometimes very vividly. Farsighted people may also see them best at this point, although their sight for form may be best at the distance.

6. SUNLIGHT

Sun-Gazing

Light is necessary to the health of the eye, and darkness is injurious to it. Eye shades, dark glasses, darkened rooms, weaken the sight and sooner or later produce inflammations. Persons with normal sight can look directly at the sun, or at the strongest artificial light, without injury or discomfort, and persons with imperfect sight are never permanently injured by such lights, though temporary ill effects, lasting from a few minutes to a few hours, days, weeks, months, or longer, may be produced. In all abnormal conditions of the eyes, light is beneficial. It is rarely sufficient to cure, but is a great help in gaining relaxation by other methods.

The quickest way to get results from the curative power of sunlight is to focus the rays with a burning glass on the white part of the eye when the patient looks far downward, moving the light from side to side to avoid heat. This may be done for part of a minute at frequent intervals.

Looking at the sun, while slower in its results, has often been sufficient to effect permanent cures, sometimes in a very short time. There is a right way and a wrong way to do this. Persons with imperfect sight should never look directly at the sun at first, because, while no permanent harm can come from it, great temporary inconvenience may result. Such persons should begin by looking to one side of the sun, and after becoming accustomed to the strong light, should look a little nearer to its source, and so on until they become able to look directly at the sun without discomfort.

Sun-Gazing

It is a well-known fact that the constant protection of the eyes from the sunlight, or from other kinds of light, is followed by weakness or inflammation of the eyes or eyelids. Children living in dark rooms, where the stuff seldom enters, acquire an intolerance for the light. Some of them keep their eyes covered with their hands, or bury their faces in a pillow and do all they possibly can to avoid exposure of their eyes to ordinary light.

I have seen many hundreds of cases of young children brought to the clinic with ulceration of the cornea, which may become sufficient to cause blindness. Putting these children in a dark room is a blunder. My best results in the cure of these cases were obtained by encouraging the patients to spend a good deal of the time out of doors, with their faces exposed to the direct rays of the sun. In a short time these children became able to play and enjoy themselves a great deal more out of doors, exposed to the sunlight, than when they protected their eyes from the light.

Not only is the sun beneficial to children with inflammation of the cornea, but it is also beneficial to adults. When the patient looks down sufficiently, the white part of the eye can be exposed by gently lifting the upper lid, while the sun's rays strike directly upon this part of the eyeball. In most cases it is possible to focus the strong light of the sun on the white part of the eyeball with the aid of a strong convex glass, being careful to move the light from side to side quite rapidly to avoid the heat. After such a treatment, the patient almost immediately becomes able to open his eyes widely in the light.

Dark Glasses Are Injurious

He was a very intelligent chauffeur, and very polite and popular with most people. I enjoyed listening to his experiences in driving various types of cars. Nothing seemed to give him so much pleasure as to get into a "jam" and get out without suffering any injury to his own car or without tearing the "enemy" apart. The "enemy," as he explained, were the numerous other cars which were driven by chauffeurs who did not understand their business very well and who enjoyed teasing the inexperienced drivers.

One day we were driving to the seashore. The sun was very bright and the reflection of the light from the sun on the water was very strong and made most of the occupants of the car very uncomfortable. Personally I enjoyed the strong light of the sun. The chauffeur did not wear glasses for the protection of his eyes from the sun or dust and I asked him if he had ever worn them. He very promptly answered me by saying that he had worn them at one time, but discontinued wearing them because he found that after wearing them for a few days, his eyes became more sensitive to the light than they were before. He said he could not understand why it was that when he wore glasses to protect his eyes from the dust he accumulated more foreign bodies in his eyes than ever before. This seemed strange to the people in the car and they asked him to explain. It was decided that when the dust got into the eyes, the glasses prevented the dust from going out.

The eyes need the light of the sun. When the sun's rays are excluded from the eyes by dark glasses, the eyes become very sensitive to the sun when the glasses are removed.

SUNLIGHT

Demonstrate

1. That sun treatment is an immediate benefit to many diseases of the eye.

Before the treatment, take a record of your best vision of the Snellen test card with both eyes together and each eye separately without glasses. Then sit in the sun with your eyes closed, slowly moving your head a short distance from side to side, and allowing the sun to shine directly on your closed eyelids. Forget about your eyes; just think of something pleasant and let your mind drift from one pleasant thought to another. Before opening your eyes, palm for a few minutes. Then test your vision of the test card and note the improvement. Get as much sun treatment as you possibly can, one, two, three or more hours daily.

When the sun is not shining, substitute a strong electric light. A 1,000 watt electric light is preferable, but requires special wiring. However, a 250 watt or 300 watt light can be used with benefit, and does not require special wiring. Sit about six inches from the light, or as near as you can without discomfort from the heat, allowing it to shine on your closed eyelids as in the sun treatment.

2. That the strong light of the sun focused on the sclera, or white part of the eyeball, with the sun glass, also improves the vision.

After the eyes have become accustomed to the sunlight with the eyes closed, focus the light of the sun on the closed eyelids with the sun glass. Move the glass rapidly from side to side while doing this for a few minutes. Then have the patient open his eyes and look as far down as possible, and in this way, the pupil is protected by the lower lid. Gently lift the upper lid, so that only the white part of the eye is exposed, as the sun's rays fall directly upon this part of the eyeball. The sun glass may now be used on the white part of the eye for a few seconds, moving it quickly from side to side and in various directions. Notice that after the use of the sun glass, the vision is improved.

7. CENTRAL FIXATION

Demonstrate

That central fixation improves the vision. The normal eye is always at rest and always has central fixation. Central fixation cannot be obtained through any effort. When an effort is made by the normal eye, central fixation is always lost. In central fixation, one sees best the point regarded while all other points are seen less clearly.

Look at the upper left hand corner of the back of a chair. Note that all other parts of the chair are not seen so well. Look at the top of a letter at a distance at which it can be seen clearly. Then quickly look at the bottom of the letter. Alternate. When the eyes go up, the letter appears to move down. Then the eyes move down, the letter appears to move up. Coincident with this movement, you can observe that you see best the point regarded and all other points less clearly or less distinctly. When you can imagine the letter to be moving, it is possible for you to see best where you are looking.

The size of the letter or object seen does not matter. Central fixation can be demonstrated with the smallest letters which are printed, or the smallest objects. Close the eyes and remember or imagine how the small letter would look if you imagined one part best. By shifting from one part of the letter to another, central fixation with the eyes closed may be made continuous for one-half minute or longer. Then with the eyes open, it is possible for one second or less to see, remember, or imagine the same small letter or other objects in the same way, - one part best.

Note that when the letters are read easily and clearly, they are always seen by central fixation, and relaxation is felt. Central fixation is a rest to the nerves and when practiced continuously, it relieves strain and improves the vision to normal.

29

Demonstrate

I. That the smaller the object regarded, the easier it is to remember. One can, with time and trouble, become able to remember all the words of one page of a book. It is easier to remember one word than all the words of a page. It is still easier to remember one letter of a word better than all the letters. Regard a capital letter. Demonstrate that it is easier to see or remember the top of the letter best, and the bottom of it less clearly than to remember the top and bottom perfectly and simultaneously. Now look directly at the upper right hand corner and imagine one-fourth of the letter best. Then cover the remaining three-quarters of the letter with a piece of paper. It is possible to look directly at the exposed part of the letter and imagine half of it best. Cover the part that is not seen distinctly, and demonstrate that half of the exposed part of the letter can be seen or imagined best, while the rest of it is not seen so clearly. With the aid of the screen, an area as small as an ordinary period, may finally be imagined. Demonstrate that the imagination of a perfectly black small period, forming part of a small letter at fifteen feet, enables one to distinguish that letter.

II. That, with the eyes closed, a small black period can be imagined blacker than one three inches in diameter. If this fact cannot be readily demonstrated with the eyes closed:

1. Stand close to a wall of a room, three feet or less, and regard a small black spot on the wall six feet from the floor. Note that you cannot see a small black spot near the bottom of the wall at the same time.

2. Place your hand on the wall six feet from the floor, and note that you cannot see your hand clearly when you look at the bottom of the wall.

8. FINE PRINT

Read Fine Print

Many nearsighted patients can read fine print or diamond type at less than ten inches from their eyes easily, perfectly and quickly, by alternately regarding the Snellen test card at different distances, from three feet up to fifteen feet or further. The vision may be improved, at first temporarily, and later, by repetition, a permanent gain usually follows.

It is a valuable fact to know, that when fine print is read perfectly, the nearsightedness or myopia disappears during this period. It can only be maintained at first for a fraction of a second, and later more continuously.

Nearsighted patients and others, with the help of the fine print can usually demonstrate that staring at a small letter always lowers the vision, and that the same fact is true when regarding distant letters or objects.

With the help of the fine print, the nearsighted patient can also demonstrate that one can remember perfectly only what has been seen perfectly; that one imagines perfectly only what is remembered perfectly, and that perfect sight is only a perfect imagination.

A great many people are very suspicious of the imagination, and feel or believe that things imagined are never true. The more ignorant the patient, the less respect do they have for their imagination, or the imagination of other people. It comes to them as a great shock, with a feeling of discomfort, to discover that the perfect imagination of a known letter improves the sight for unknown letters of the Snellen test card, or for other objects.

It is a fact, that one can read fine print perfectly, with perfect relaxation, with great relief to eyestrain, pain fatigue and discomfort, not only of the eyes, but of all other nerves of the body.

Fine Print A Benefit To The Eye

Seven Truths of Normal Sight
1—Normal Sight can always be demonstrated in the normal eye, but only under favorable condition.
2—Central Fixation: The letter or part of the letter regarded is always seen best.
3—Shifting: The point regarded changes rapidly and continuously.
4—Swinging: When the shifting is slow, the letters appear to move from side to side, or in other directions, with a pendulum-like motion.
5—Memory is perfect. The color and background of the letters, or other objects seen, are remembered perfectly, instantaneously and continuously.
6—Imagination is good. One may even see the white part of letters whiter than it really is, while the black is not altered by distance, illumination, size, or form, of the letters.
7—Rest or relaxation of the eye and mind is perfect and can always be demonstrated.
When one of these seven fundamentals is perfect, all are perfect.

It is impossible to read fine print without relaxing. Therefore the reading of such print, contrary to what is generally believed, is a great benefit to the eyes. Persons who can read perfectly fine print, like the above specimen, are relieved of pain and fatigue while they are doing it, and this relief is often permanent.

Persons who cannot read it are benefited by observing its blackness, and remembering it with the eyes open and closed alternately. By bringing the print so near to the eyes that it cannot be read pain is sometimes relieved instantly, because when the patient realizes that there is no possibility of reading it the eyes do not try to do so. In myopia, however, it is sometimes a benefit to strain to read fine print.

Persons who can read fine print perfectly imagine that they see between the lines streaks of white whiter than the margin of the page, and persons who cannot read it also see these streaks, but not so well. When the patient becomes able to increase the vividness of these appearances* the sight always improves.

* See Halos on page 24.

Relaxation From Fine Print

A business card, 3" x 2" with fine print on one side is held in front of the eyes as near as possible, the upper part in contact with the eye-brows, the lower part resting lightly on the nose.

The patient looks directly at the fine print without trying to see. Being so close to the eyes most people realize that it is impossible to read the fine print and do not try, in this way they obtain a measure of relaxation which is sufficient to benefit the sight very much.

The patient moves the card from side to side a short distance slowly and sees the card moving provided the movement is not too short or too slow. The shorter the movement and the slower it is, the better.

Some patients, although the card is held very close, note that the white spaces between the lines become whiter and the black letters become blacker and clearer. In some cases one or more words of the fine print will be seen in flashes or even continuously as long as no effort is made to see or to read the fine print.

This movement of the card should be kept up to obtain the best results, for many hours every day. The hand which holds the card may soon become fatigued; one may then use the hands alternately. Some patients vary this by holding the card with both hands at the same time.

The amount of light is not important.

Relaxation From Fine Print
A business card, 3" x 2" with fine print on one side is held in front of the eyes as near as possible, the upper part in contact with the eye-brows, the lower part resting lightly on the nose.

The patient looks directly at the fine print without trying to see. Being so close to the eyes most people realize that it is impossible to read the fine print and do not try, in this way they obtain a measure of relaxation which is sufficient to benefit the sight very much.

The patient moves the card from side to side a short distance slowly and sees the card moving provided the movement is not too short or too slow. The shorter the movement and the slower it is, the better.

Some patients, although the card is held very close, note that the white spaces between the lines become whiter and the black letters become blacker and clearer. In some cases one or more words of the fine print will be seen in flashes or even continuously as long as no effort is made to see or to read the fine print.

This movement of the card should be kept up to obtain the best results, for many hours every day. The hand which holds the card may soon become fatigued; one may then use the hands alternately. Some patients vary this by holding the card with both hands at the same time.

The amount of light is not important.

W.H. Bates, M.D.   Bates Method Nuggets   www.VisionsOfJoy.org

9. ATTITUDE

Optimism

Optimism is a great help in obtaining a cure of imperfect sight. About ten years ago a patient was treated for cataract, complicated with glaucoma. After two weeks of daily treatment the vision improved very much and the patient became able to travel about the streets without a companion to guide her. Her vision at this time had improved from perception of light to 10/200. After palming, swinging, and the memory of perfect sight, her vision was still further improved. She was very much encouraged and returned home full of enthusiasm to carry out the treatment to the very best of her ability.

Soon afterwards things did not go well at home. The patient became very much depressed and stopped her daily practice. Her daughter was very enthusiastic, and realized that her mother had been very materially improved and that further treatment would bring about a complete cure. She talked to her mother for half an hour or more and encouraged her to continue with her practice. The patient responded favorably, got busy, and was able to bring back much of the sight which had been lost. She made further improvement every day.

At times the mother was very pessimistic. She was continually complaining that she knew very well that she would never get her sight back. Then the daughter would start in with her optimism.

One bright, sunshiny morning the mother got up, took a card with diamond type printed on one side, and was greatly surprised to read it without any trouble. In three months her distant vision was normal.

Fear

Nearsighted people have frequently been told that it is necessary for them to wear glasses constantly, to prevent their eyes from becoming worse. They are afraid that this statement may be true, and one cannot blame them for hesitating to leave their glasses off permanently.

One of my patients stated that she suffered very much from headaches. They were so severe that they made her ill, and confined her to her bed at least once a week. While wearing her glasses, she still was in pain, but was afraid, if she left them off, the headaches would become worse. By discarding her glasses, practicing palming, swinging, and the memory of perfect sight, her eyes and head improved immediately. When she resumed her glasses again, she at once became uncomfortable, and the pain returned. She decided to leave them off permanently, and her headaches disappeared.

Some years ago an optician consulted me about his headaches. When I examined his glasses, I found that they were plane window glass. He said that when he wore them his headaches were better, but his wife confided to me that this was not true. He was troubled more when he wore them. He was suffering from fear.

I saw him again a year later and learned that he had permanently discarded his glasses, at my suggestion, during all that time, and was free of headaches.

It has been a habit with me, when patients who suffer from fear of the consequences that might happen if they did not wear their glasses, to have them demonstrate the facts. When the truth is known, fear is abolished. It is very easy in most cases to teach patients some of the causes of headaches.

Think Right

"As a man thinketh in his heart so is he," is a saying which is invariably true when the sight is concerned. When a person remembers or imagines an object of sight perfectly the sight is perfect; when he remembers it imperfectly the sight is imperfect. The idea that to do anything well requires effort, ruins the sight of many children and adults; for every thought of effort in the mind produces an error of refraction in the eye. The idea that large objects are easier to see than small ones results in the failure to see small objects. The fear that light will hurt the eyes actually produces sensitiveness to light. To demonstrate the truth of these statements is a great benefit.

Remember a letter or other object perfectly, and note that the sight is improved and pain and fatigue relieved; remember the object imperfectly, and note that the vision is lowered, while pain and fatigue may be produced or increased.

Rest the eyes by closing or palming, and note that the vision is improved, and pain and discomfort relieved; stare at a letter, concentrate upon it, make an effort to see it, and note that it disappears, and that a feeling of discomfort or pain is produced.

Note that a small part of a large object is seen better than the rest of it.

Accustom the eyes to strong light; learn to look at the sun; note that the vision is not lowered but improved, and that the light causes less and less discomfort.

Remember your successes (things seen perfectly); forget your failures (things seen imperfectly); patients who do this are cured quickly.

Brain Tension

The brain has many nerves. Part of these nerves are called ganglion cells and originate in some particular part of the brain. Each has a function of its own. They are connected with other ganglion cells and with the aid of nerve fibres are connected with others located in various parts of the brain as well as in the spinal cord, the eye, the ear, the nerves of smell, taste, and the nerves of touch. The function of each ganglion cell of the brain is different from that of all others. When the ganglion cells are healthy, they function in a normal manner.

The retina of the eye contains numerous ganglion cells which regulate special things such as normal vision, normal memory, normal imagination and they do this with a control more or less accurate of other ganglion cells of the whole body. The retina has a similar structure to parts of the brain. It is connected to the brain by the optic nerve.

Many nerves from the ganglion cells of the retina carry conscious and unconscious control of other ganglion cells which are connected to other parts of the body.

When the ganglion cells are diseased or at fault, the functions of all parts of the body are not normally maintained. In all cases of imperfect sight, it has been repeatedly demonstrated that the ganglion cells and nerves of the brain are under a strain. When this strain is corrected by treatment, the functions of the ganglion and other cells become normal. The importance of the mental treatment cannot be over-estimated.

A study of the facts has demonstrated that a disease of some ganglion in any part of the body occurs in a similar ganglion in the brain.

Brain tension of one or more nerves always means disease of the nerve ganglia. Treatment of the mind with the aid of the sight, memory and imagination has cured many cases of imperfect sight without other treatment.

10. MEMORY & IMAGINATION

Demonstrate

That memory and imagination improve the vision.

Look at the large letter at the top of the card and note that it may be more or less blurred. Close the eyes and remember or imagine the same letter perfectly. Then open both eyes and imagine it as well as you can. In a second or less, close your eyes and remember the letter perfectly. When this is accomplished open the eyes and imagine it as well as you can. Close them quickly after a second or less. Practice the slow, short, easy swing and alternately remember the large letter with the eyes closed for part of a minute or longer, and then open the eyes and imagine it as well as you can.

When done properly, you will be able to improve your vision of the large letter until it becomes quite perfect. Then practice in the same way with the first letter of the second line. Improve your imagination of the first letter of the second line in flashes, until it improves sufficiently for you to recognize the next letter without looking at it.

Improve the sight of the first letter of each line by alternately remembering it with the eyes closed for part of a minute and then flashing it for just a moment, a second or less. You should be told what the first letter of each line is. With your eyes closed remember it as perfectly as you can. Then open your eyes and test your imagination for the letter for a very short time, one second or even less. Keep your eyes closed for at least a part of a minute, while remembering the known letter. The flashes of the known letter with the eyes open become more frequent and last longer, until you become able to see, not only the known letter, but other unknown letters on the same line.

The Memory Cure

When the sight is perfect, the memory is also perfect, because the mind is perfectly relaxed. Therefore the sight may be improved by any method that improves the memory. The easiest thing to remember is a small black spot of no particular size and form; but when the sight is imperfect it will be found impossible to remember it with the eyes open and looking at letters, or other objects with definite outlines. It may, however, be remembered for a few seconds or longer, when the eyes are closed and covered, or when looking at a blank surface where there is nothing particular to see.

By cultivating the memory under these favorable conditions, it gradually becomes possible to retain it under unfavorable ones, that is, when the eyes are open and the mind conscious of the impressions of sight. By alternately remembering the period with the eyes closed and covered and then looking at the Snellen test card, or other letters or objects; or by remembering it when looking away from the card where there is nothing particular to see, and then looking back; the patient becomes able, in a longer or shorter time, to retain the memory when looking at the card, and thus becomes able to read the letters with normal vision.

Many children have been cured very quickly by this method. Adults who have worn glasses have greater difficulty. Even under favorable conditions, the period cannot be remembered for more than a few seconds, unless one shifts from one part of it to another. One can also shift from one period, or other small black object, to another.

The Imagination Cure

When the imagination is perfect the mind is always perfectly relaxed, and as it is impossible to relax and imagine a letter perfectly, and at the same time strain and see it imperfectly, it follows that when one imagines that one sees a letter perfectly one actually does see it, as demonstrated by the retinoscope, no matter how great an error of refraction the eye may previously have had. The sight, therefore, may often be improved very quickly by the aid of the imagination. To use this method the patient may proceed as follows:

Look at a letter at the distance at which it is seen best. Close and cover the eyes so as to exclude all the light, and remember it. Do this alternately until the memory is nearly equal to the sight. Next, after remembering the letter with the eyes closed and covered, and while still holding the mental picture of it, look at a blank surface a foot or more to the side of it, at the distance at which you wish to see it.

Again close and cover the eyes and remember the letter, and on opening them look a little nearer to it. Gradually reduce the distance between the point of fixation and the letter, until able to look directly at it and imagine it as well as it is remembered with the eyes closed and covered. The letter will then be seen perfectly, and other letters in its neighborhood will come out. If unable to remember the whole letter, you may be able to imagine a black period as forming part of it. If you can do this, the letter will also be seen perfectly.

How To Improve The Sight By Means Of The Imagination

Remember the letter o in diamond type [ₒ] with the eyes closed and covered. If you are able to do this, it will appear to have a short, slow swing, less than its own diameter.

Look at an unknown letter on the test card which you can see only as a gray spot, at ten feet or more, and imagine that it has a swing of not more than a quarter of an inch.

Imagine the top of the unknown letter to be straight, still maintaining the swing. If this is in accordance with the fact, the swing will be unchanged. If it is not, the swing will become uneven, or longer, or will be lost.

If the swing is altered, try another guess. If you can't tell the difference between two guesses, it is because the swing is too long. Palm and remember the o with its short swing, and you may become able to shorten that of the larger letter.

In this way you can ascertain, without seeing the letter, whether its four sides are straight, curved, or open. You may then be able to imagine the whole letter. This is easiest with the eyes closed and covered. If the swing is modified, you will know that you have made a mistake. In that case repeat from the beginning.

When you get the right letter imagine it alternately with the eyes closed and open, until you are able to imagine it as well when you look at it as when your eyes are closed and covered. In that case you will actually see the letter.

How To Improve The Sight By Means Of The Imagination: No. 2

In a recent issue directions were given for improving the vision by the aid of the imagination. According to this method the patient ascertains what a letter is by imagining each of the four sides to be straight, curved, or open, and noting the effect of each guess upon the imagined swing of the letter. Another method which has succeeded even better with many patients is to judge the correctness of the guess by observing its effect on the appearance of the letter.

Look at a letter which can be seen only as a gray spot, and imagine the top is straight. If the guess is right, the spot will probably become blacker; if it is wrong, the spot may become fainter or disappear. If no difference is apparent, rest the eyes by looking away, closing, or palming, and try again.

In many cases, when one side has been imagined correctly, the whole letter will come out. If it does not, proceed to imagine the other sides as above directed. If, when all four sides have been imagined correctly, a letter does not come out, palm and repeat.

One can even bring out a letter that one cannot see at all in this way. Look at a line of letters which cannot be seen, and imagine the top of the first letter to be straight. If the guess is correct, the line may become apparent, and by continued practice the letter may come out clearly enough to be distinguished.

Test Your Imagination!

With the eyes closed remember some letter, as, for example, a small letter o. Imagine the white center to be white as snow with the sun shining on it. Now open the eyes, look at the Snellen Test Card and imagine the white snow as well as you can for a few moments only; without noting so much the clearness of the letters on the card as your ability to imagine the snow white center, alternating as before with the Snellen Card.

Another method: With the eyes closed, remember and imagine as well as you can the first letter, which should be known, on each line of the Snellen Test Card, beginning with the larger letters. Then open your eyes and imagine the same letter for a few moments only, alternating until the known letter is imagined sufficiently well that the second letter is seen without any effort on your part.

Third method: With the eyes closed remember or imagine a small black period for part of a minute or longer. Then with the eyes open, looking at no object in particular and without trying to see, imagine in your mind the black period. Should you believe that your vision is improved, dodge it, look somewhere else. This you can practice at all times, in all places, at your work as well as when sitting quietly in your room practicing with the Snellen Test Card. When the period is imagined perfectly with the eyes open, one cannot dodge perfect sight, which comes without any effort whatsoever.

Demonstrate

That vision is always imagination, either perfect or imperfect. What we see is only what we think or imagine we see. The white center of the letter "O", when seen perfectly, appears to be whiter than it really is, or whiter than the rest of the card. That part of the center of the "O" which is in contact with the black appears to be the whitest part of the white center. By covering the black part of the "O" with a screen, which has an opening in the center, the whiteness of the center of the "O" appears to be the same shade of white as the rest of the card. Now, remove the screen, and at the first glance the center of the "O" appears for a short time to be much whiter than it really is.

In other words, one sees something which is not really seen, but only imagined. When some people enter a room which is totally dark, they often imagine that they see a white ghost. They don't really see it; they only imagine it, but their imagination may be so vivid that no amount of argument will convince them that they did not see the ghost.

When one looks at the upper right hand corner of a large letter of the Snellen test card, it is possible to see that point best, and all the rest of the letter not so black. The part seen best appears blacker than it really is. The part seen worse appears less black than it really is. Things seen more perfectly than they really are, are not seen, but imagined. Things seen less perfectly than they really are, are not seen imperfectly but are imagined imperfectly.

44

Demonstrate

That by practicing you can imagine a letter at ten feet as well as you can see it at one foot. Regard a letter of the Snellen test card at a distance where it cannot be readily distinguished and appears blurred. Now look at the same letter on a card at the near point, one foot or less, where it can be seen perfectly. Then close your eyes and with your finger draw the same letter in the air as well as you can remember it.

Open your eyes and continue to draw the imaginary letter with your finger while looking for only a few seconds at the blurred letter on the card at ten feet. Then close your eyes again and remember the letter well enough to draw the letter perfectly in your imagination with your finger.

Alternate drawing the letter at ten feet in your imagination with your eyes open and drawing it with your eyes closed as well as you see it at one foot or nearer. When you can draw the letter as perfectly as you remember it, you see the letter on the distant card in flashes.

By repetition you will become able not only to always imagine the known letter correctly, but to actually see it for a few seconds at a time. You cannot see a letter perfectly unless you see one part best, central fixation. Note that you obtain central fixation while practicing this method, i.e., you see one part best. Drawing the letter with your finger in your imagination enables you to follow the finger in forming the letter, and with the help of your memory, you can imagine each side of the letter best, in turn, as it is formed. By this method the memory and the imagination are improved, and when the imagination becomes perfect, the sight is perfect. You can cure the highest degrees of myopia, hypermetropia, astigmatism, atrophy of the optic nerve, cataract, glaucoma, detachment of the retina and other diseases by this method.

Demonstrate

Demonstrate that perfect sight is accomplished when the imagination is good, and that you see only what you imagine you see.

Take a Snellen test card and hold it at a distance from your eyes at which your sight is fairly good. Look at the white center of the large "O" and compare the whiteness of the center of the "O" with the whiteness of the rest of the card. You may do it readily; but if not, use a screen, that is, a card with a small hole in it. With that card, cover over the black part of the letter "O" and note the white center of the letter which is exposed by the opening in the screen. Remove the screen and observe that there is a change in the appearance of the white, which appears to be a whiter white, when the black part of the letter is exposed. When the black part of the letter is covered with a screen, the center of the "O" is of the same whiteness as the rest of the card.

It is, therefore, possible to demonstrate that you do not see the white center of the "O" whiter than the rest of the card, because you are seeing something that is not there. When you see something that is not there, you do not really see it, you only imagine it. The whiter you can imagine the center of the "O," the better becomes the vision for the letter "O," and when the vision of the letter "O" improves, the vision of all the letters on the card improves. The perfect imagination of the white center of the "O" means perfect imagination of the black, because you cannot imagine the white perfectly, without imagining the black perfectly.

By practice you may become able to imagine the letter "O" much better than it really is, and when this is accomplished, you become able to actually see unknown letters.

11. MENTAL PICTURES

Mental Pictures

Many patients with imperfect sight complain that when they close their eyes to remember a white card with black letters, they usually fail and remember instead a black card with white letters. The vision of these patients is very much improved when they become able to remember a white card white, with the black letters remembered perfectly black. Imperfect memory, imperfect imagination, imperfect sight are all caused by strain.

One patient could not remember a white pillow, but by first regarding the pillow and seeing one corner best and all the other corners worse and shifting from one comer to another he became able, when closing his eyes, to remember one comer in turn best, and obtained a good mental picture of the whole pillow. One cannot see a pillow perfectly without Central Fixation. To have Central Fixation requires relaxation or rest.

One patient who could not remember a large letter C of the Snellen Test Card, with the eyes closed, was able to remember the colors of some flowers, and then he was able to remember a letter C. In order to remember a desired mental picture one should remember perfectly some other things. This is a relaxation which helps to remember the mental picture desired. It is well to keep in mind that one cannot remember one thing perfectly and something else imperfectly at the same time.

In my book is described the case of a woman with imperfect sight who could remember a yellow buttercup with the eyes closed, perfectly, but with her eyes open and regarding the Snellen Card with imperfect sight, she had no memory of the yellow buttercup.

Mental Pictures

With imperfect sight, a mental picture of one known letter of the Snellen test card is seldom or never remembered, imagined, or seen perfectly when regarded with the eyes open. By closing the eyes, the same mental picture may be imagined more perfectly. By alternately imagining the known letter as well as possible; with the eyes open and then remembering it better with the eyes closed, the imagination improves the vision and unknown letters are seen with the eyes open.

The improvement of the vision is due to a lessening of the organic changes in the eye. When the imperfect sight is caused by opacities of the cornea, a mental picture imagined clearly lessens or cures the disease of the cornea. A large number of cases of cataract in which the lens is more or less opaque have been benefited or cured by the imagination of mental pictures. Nearly all organic changes in the eyeball which lower the vision have been improved to some extent in a few minutes; by devoting a sufficient amount of time, all organic changes in the eyeball, no matter what the cause may be, are benefited or cured by a perfect imagination of a letter, a tree, a flower, or anything which is remembered perfectly.

I do not know of any method of obtaining relaxation or perfect sight which is as efficient and certain as the imagination of mental pictures. It should be emphasized that a good or perfect imagination of mental pictures has in all cases brought about a measure of improvement which is convincing that the imagination is capable of relieving organic changes in the eye more quickly, more thoroughly, more permanently, than any other method.

How To Obtain Mental Pictures

Look at a letter on the Snellen test card.

Remember its blackness.

Shift the attention from one part of this spot of black to another. It should appear to move in a direction contrary to the imagined movement.

If it does not, try to imagine it stationary. If you succeed in doing this it will blur, or disappear. Having demonstrated that it is impossible to imagine the spot stationary, it may become possible to imagine it moving.

Having become able to form a mental picture of a black spot with the eyes closed, try to do the same with the eyes open. Alternate till the mental vision with the eyes closed and open is the same.

Having become able to imagine a black spot try to imagine the letter o in diamond type [ₒ] with the center as white as snow. Do this alternately with eyes closed and open.

If you cannot hold the picture of a letter or period commit to memory a number of letters on the test card and recite them to yourself while imagining that the card is moving.

If some other color or object is easier to imagine than a black spot it will serve the purpose equally well.

A few exceptional people may get better results with the eyes open than when they are closed.

12. THE PERIOD

The Period

The perfect memory or imagination of a period is a cure for imperfect sight. Only the color needs to be remembered. The size is immaterial, but a small period is remembered with more relaxation than a large one. It is true, however, that with perfect sight, one has the ability to remember all things perfectly.

One cannot remember a period perfectly by any kind of an effort. It usually happens that one may remember a period for a time, and then lose it by an effort. To remember a period stationary, is impossible. One has to shift more or less frequently in order to remember one period perfectly all the time, or one has to imagine the period to be moving, or one has to remember the period by central fixation, - one part best. By shifting, is meant to look away from the period and then back, but to do it so quickly that it is possible to remember the period continuously, although you are not looking at it all the time, - this with the eyes closed. Every time you blink, you shift your eyes.

You can blink so rapidly that it is not noticeable. When you close your eyes and remember a period, you cannot remember it unless you are, with your eyes closed, going through the process as though you were blinking, looking away from it and back again, but so quickly that it seems as though you were looking at the period continuously.

You cannot remember the whole of the period at once. No matter how small the period is, you cannot see or remember it perfectly, all parts equally well at the same time. You cannot remember the period perfectly by any kind of an effort. When the memory of the period is perfect, the mental and physical efficiency is increased. A perfect memory of the period does not necessarily mean that one should think only of the period.

The Period

Many people have difficulty in obtaining a mental picture of a small black period. They may try to see it by an effort which always fails. They may persist in their efforts to see or remember it, paying little or no attention to their failures or the cause of their failures. As long as they continue to strain by trying to see, they will always fail; the period becomes more indistinct.

A small black period is very readily seen. There is no letter, no figure, no object of any kind which can be obtained more easily. Demonstrate that an effort to see a small black period by staring, concentrating, trying to see, always makes it worse. Rest, relaxation, the swing, shifting, are all a great help.

Practice with a large black letter. Imagine that the upper right corner has a small black period. Do the same with other parts of the large letter. This practice will enable you to understand central fixation, seeing best where you are looking. Central fixation can always be demonstrated when the sight is good. When the sight is poor or imperfect, central fixation is absent.

The benefits which can be obtained from the use of the period are very numerous. A perfect memory can only be obtained when the sight is perfect. A perfect imagination can only be obtained when the sight and the memory are perfect. The period is the smallest letter or other object which is perfect or becomes perfect by perfect memory or perfect imagination.

•   •   •   •   •   .   .

The Colon

While the colon is a valuable punctuation mark, it has a very unusual and better use in helping the memory, imagination, and sight. Medium sized or small letters at the distance are improved promptly by the proper use of the colon. While the eyes are closed or open, the top period should be imagined best while the lower period is more or less blurred and not seen so well. In a few moments it is well to shift and imagine the lower period best while the upper period is imagined not so well. Common sense makes it evident that one period cannot be imagined best unless there is some other period or other object which is seen worse. The smallest colon that can be imagined is usually the one that is imagined more readily than a larger colon.

When palming, swinging, et cetera, cannot be practiced sufficiently well to obtain improvement in the eyesight, the memory or imagination of the small colon, one part best, can usually be practiced with benefit. To remember or imagine a colon perfectly requires constant shifting. When the colon is remembered or imagined perfectly, and this cannot be done by any effort or strain, the sight is always improved and the memory and imagination are also improved.

It is interesting to note that the smaller the colon, the blacker and better can one remember, imagine, or see one period of it, with benefit to the sight. One may feel that the memory of a very small colon should be more difficult than the memory of a large one, but strange to say it can be demonstrated in most cases that the very small colon is remembered best. If the movement of the colon is absent, the sight is always imperfect. In other words, it requires a stare, strain, and effort to make the colon stop its apparent motion.

: : : : : : :

13. SHIFTING

Shifting

When the normal eye has normal sight it is at rest and when it is at rest it is always moving or shifting. Shifting may be done consciously with improvement in the vision, or it may be done unconsciously with impaired vision.

Shifting can be practiced correctly and incorrectly. A wrong way to shift is to turn the head to the right while the eyes are turned to the left, or to turn the head to the left while the eyes are turned to the right.

To improve imperfect sight by shifting, it is well to move the head and eyes so far away that the first letter or object imagined is too far away to be seen at all clearly. Shifting from small letters to large letters alternately may be a greater benefit than shifting from one small letter to another small letter.

Quite frequently the vision is decidedly improved by shifting continuously from one side of a small letter to the other side, while the letter is imagined to be moving in the opposite direction. When the shifting is slow, short, and easy, the best results in the improvement in the vision are obtained. Any attempt to stop the shifting always lowers the vision. The letter or other object which appeared to move is usually shifting a short distance—one half or one quarter of an inch. It is not possible to imagine any particular letter or other object stationary for a longer time than one minute.

While the patient is seated, benefit can be obtained from shifting, but even more benefit can be obtained when the shifting is practiced while the patient is standing and moving the head and shoulders, in fact the whole body, a very short distance from side to side. Shifting the whole body makes it easier to shift a short distance and may explain why this method is best.

The Easy Shift

Some time ago a man came to me for treatment of his eyes. Without glasses his vision was about one-half of the normal. This patient could not palm without suffering an agony of pain and depression. He had pain in different parts of his body as well as in his eyes and the pain was usually very severe. The long swing, the short swing tired him exceedingly and made his sight worse. I asked him to tell me what there was that he could remember which caused him no discomfort.

He said, "Everything that I see disturbs me if I make an effort." "I try very hard not to make an effort, but the harder I try the worse do I feel."

When he could not practice palming, swinging or memory successfully I suggested to him that he look from one side of the room to the other, paying no attention to what he saw, but to remember as well as he could a room in his home. For two hours he practiced this and was able to move his eyes from one side of the room to the other without paying any attention to the things that were moving or to the things he saw. This was a rest to him, and when his vision was tested, much to my surprise, he read the Snellen Test Card with normal vision at twenty feet. I handed him some diamond type, which he read without difficulty and without his glasses.

Since that time I have had other patients who were unable to remember or imagine things without straining and they usually obtained marked benefit by practicing the EASY SHIFT.

No one can obtain perfect sight without constantly shifting, easily, without effort. THE EASY SHIFT is easy because it is done without trying to remember, to imagine or to see. As soon as one makes an effort the shift becomes difficult and no benefit is obtained.

Demonstrate

1. Demonstrate that when the eyes are stationary, they are under a tremendous strain. Stand before the Snellen test card at a distance of fifteen or twenty feet. Look directly at one small area of a large letter, which can be seen clearly. Stare at that part of the letter without closing the eyes and without shifting the eyes to some other point. The vision becomes worse and the letter blurs. Stare continuously, and note that the longer you stare, the more difficult it is to keep the eyes focused on that one point or part of the letter. Not only does the stare become more difficult, but the eyes become tired; and by making a greater effort, the eyes pain, or a headache is produced. The stare can cause fatigue of the whole body when the effort is sufficiently strong and prolonged.

2. Demonstrate that when the eyes are moving from one point to another, frequently, easily and continuously, the stare, the strain, or the effort to see is prevented and the eyes feel rested. In fact, the eyes are not at rest except when they are moving. Note that when you look at a letter on the Snellen test card and alternately shift from the top to the bottom of it, the vision remains good or is improved. When the letter is seen perfectly, the eyes are shifting; and when seen imperfectly, the shifting stops.

3. Close your eyes and remember your signature. This can usually be done quite perfectly. Try to remember the first and the last letter of your name simultaneously. This is an impossible thing to do and requires a strain. If you shift from one letter to another, you can remember your signature, one letter at a time; but if you make an effort to remember it, the memory and the imagination of your signature disappears.

14. SEE THINGS MOVING

See Things Moving

When the sight is perfect the subject is able to observe that all objects regarded appear to be moving. A letter seen at the near point or at the distance appears to move slightly in various directions. The pavement comes toward one in walking, and the houses appear to move in a direction opposite to one's own. In reading the page appears to move in a direction opposite to that of the eye. If one tries to imagine things stationary, the vision is at once lowered and discomfort and pain may be produced, not only in the eyes and head, but in other parts of the body.

This movement is usually so slight that it is seldom noticed till the attention is called to it, but it may be so conspicuous as to be plainly observable even to persons with markedly imperfect sight. If such persons, for instance, hold the hand within six inches of the face and turn the head and eyes rapidly from side to side, the hand will be seen to move in a direction opposite to that of the eyes. If it does not move, it will be found that the patient is straining to see it in the eccentric field. By observing this movement it becomes possible to see or imagine a less conspicuous movement, and thus the patient may gradually become able to observe a slight movement in every object regarded. Some persons with imperfect sight have been cured simply by imagining that they see things moving all day long.

The world moves. Let it move. All objects move if you let them. Do not interfere with this movement, or try to stop it. This cannot be done without an effort which impairs the efficiency of the eye and mind.

See Things Moving

When riding in a railroad train, travelling rapidly, a passenger looking out a window can imagine more or less vividly that stationary objects, trees, houses, telegraph poles, are moving past in the opposite direction. If one walks along the street, objects to either side appear to be moving. When the eyes move from side to side a long distance with or without the movement of the head or body it is possible to imagine objects not directly regarded to be moving. To see things moving avoid looking directly at them while moving the eyes.

The Long Swing: No matter how great the mental or other strain may be, one can, by moving the eyes a long distance from side to side with the movement of the head and body in the same direction, imagine things moving opposite over a wide area. The eyes or mind are benefitted.

The Short Swing: To imagine things are moving a quarter of an inch or less, gradually shorten the long swing and decrease the speed to a rate of a second or less for each swing. Another method is to remember a small letter perfectly with the eyes closed and noting the short swing. Alternate with the eyes open and closed.

The Universal Swing: Demonstrate that when one imagines or sees one letter on a card at a distance or at a near point that the card moves with the letter and that every other letter or object seen or imagined in turn also swings. This is the universal swing. Practice it all the time because the ability to see or to do other things is benefitted.

Practice the imagination of the swing constantly. If one imagines things are stationary, the vision is always imperfect, and effort is required and one does not feel comfortable. To stare and strain takes time. To let things move is easier. One should plan to practice the swing observed by the eye with normal vision: as short at least as the width of the letter at twenty feet or six inches, as slow as a second to each movement and all done easily, rhythmically, continuously.

Moving

The world moves. Let it move. People are moving all day long. It is normal, right, proper that they should move. Just try to keep your head, or one finger, one toe, stationary, or keep your eyes open continuously. If you try to stare at a small letter or a part of it without blinking, note what happens. Most people who have tried it discover that the mind wanders, the vision becomes less, pain and fatigue are produced.

Stand facing a window and note the relative position of a curtain cord to the background. Take a long step to the right. Observe that the background has become different. Now take a long step to the left. The background has changed again. Avoid regarding the curtain cord. While moving from side to side, it is possible to imagine the cord moving in the opposite direction. By practice one becomes able to imagine stationary objects not seen to be moving as continuously, as easily, as objects in the field of vision.

Universal Swing: When one becomes able to imagine all objects seen, remembered, or imagined, to be moving with a slow, short, easy swing, this is called the Universal Swing. It is a very desirable thing to have, because when it is imagined with the eyes closed or open, one cannot simultaneously imagine pain, fatigue, or imperfect sight.

The Universal Swing can be obtained without one being conspicuous. With the hand covered, move the thumb from side to side about one-quarter of an inch, and move the eyes with the thumb. Stationary objects can be imagined to be moving.

When walking rapidly forward, the floor or the sidewalk appears to move backward. It is well to be conscious of this imagined movement.

Never imagine stationary objects to be stationary. To do this, is a strain, a strain which lowers the vision.

Dizziness

Dizziness is caused by eyestrain. Some people when standing on the roof of a house looking down, strain their eyes and become dizzy. Usually the dizziness is produced unconsciously. It can be produced consciously, however, by staring or straining to see some distant or near object.

Some persons when riding in an elevator are always dizzy and may suffer from attacks of imperfect sight with headache, nausea, and other nervous discomforts. An old lady, aged sixty, told me that riding in an elevator always made her dizzy, and produced headaches with pain in her eyes and head. I tested her vision and found it to be normal both for distance and for reading without glasses. To obtain some facts, I rode in an elevator with her from the top to the bottom of the building and back again. I watched her eyes closely and found that she was staring at the floors which appeared to be moving opposite to the movement of the elevator. I asked her the question: "Why do you stare at the floors which appear to be moving by?"

She answered: "I do not like to see them move, and I am trying to correct the illusion by making an effort to keep them stationary. The harder I try, the worse I feel."

I suggested to her that she look at one part of the elevator and avoid looking at the floors. Her discomfort was at once relieved, and she was soon cured.

In all cases of dizziness, the stare or strain is always evident. When the stare or strain is relieved or prevented, dizziness does not occur.

With advancing years attacks of dizziness and blindness occur more frequently than in younger individuals. All attacks of dizziness with blindness are quite readily cured by practicing the imagination of the swing, the memory of perfect sight, or by palming.

How Not To Concentrate

To remember the letter o of diamond type [o] continuously and without effort proceed as follows:

Imagine a little black spot on the right-hand side of the o blacker than the rest of the letter; then imagine a similar spot on the left-hand side. Shift the attention from the right-hand period to the left, and observe that every time that you think of the left period the o appears to move to the right, and every time you think of the right one it appears to move to the left. This motion, when the shifting is done properly, is very short, less than the width of the letter. Later you may become able to imagine the o without conscious shifting and swinging, but whenever the attention is directed to the matter these things will be noticed.

Now do the same with a letter on the test card. If the shifting is normal, it will be noted that the letter can be regarded indefinitely, and that it appears to have a slight motion.

To demonstrate that the attempt to concentrate spoils the memory, or imagination, and the vision:

Try to think continuously of a period on one part of an imagined letter. The period and the whole letter will soon disappear. Or try to imagine two or more periods, or the whole letter, equally black and distinct at one time. This will be found to be even more difficult.

Do the same with a letter on the test card. The results will be the same.

Try Dancing

There has been repeatedly published in this magazine and in my book that the imagination of stationary objects to be moving is a rest and relaxation and a benefit to the sight. Young children, when one or both eyes turn in or out, are benefited by having them swing from side to side with a regular rhythmical motion. This motion prevents the stare and the strain and improves the appearance of the eyes.

It helps the sight of most children to play puss-in-the-corner or to play hide-and-seek. Children become very much excited and laugh and carry on and have a good time and it certainly is a benefit to their sight. It seems to me that these children would be benefited by going to dancing school.

Many of my patients practice the long swing in the office and give strangers the impression that they are practicing steps of a dance. One patient with imperfect sight from detachment of the retina recently told me over the telephone that he went to a dance the night before and although he lost considerable sleep his sight was very much improved on the following morning.

Dancing is certainly a great help to keep things moving or to imagine stationary objects are moving, and is always recommended. Some people have told me that the memory of the music, the constant rhythmic motion and the relaxation have improved the vision.

Demonstrate

That the eyes can be used correctly or incorrectly when walking.

Many people have complained that after walking a short distance slowly, easily and without any special effort, they become nervous, tired and their eyes feel the symptoms and consequences of strain. When they were taught the correct way to use their eyes while walking, the symptoms of fatigue or strain disappeared.

The facts can be demonstrated with the aid of a straight line on the floor or the seam in the carpet.

Stand with the right foot to the right of the line and the left foot to the left of the line. Now put your right foot forward and look to the left of the line. Then put your left foot forward and look to the right of the line. When you walk forward, look to the left of the line when your right foot moves forward. Look to the right of the line when your left foot moves forward. Note that it is difficult to do this longer than a few seconds without uncertainty, discomfort, pain, headache, dizziness or nausea.

Now practice the right method of walking and using the eyes. When the right foot moves forward, look to the right; and when the left foot moves forward, look to the left. Note that the straight line seems to sway in the direction opposite to the movement of the eyes and foot, i.e., when the eyes and foot move to the right, the line seems to move to the left. When the eyes and foot move to the left, the line seems to move to the right. Note that this is done easily, without any hesitation or discomfort.

When you walk, you can imagine that you are looking at the right foot as you step forward with that foot. When you step forward with the left foot, you can imagine that you are looking at your left foot. This can be done in a slow walk or quite rapidly while running straight ahead or in a circle.

15. SWAYING

Swaying

It is a great help in the improving of vision to have the patient demonstrate that staring at one part of a letter at ten feet or further is a difficult thing to do for any length of time without lowering the vision and producing pain, discomfort, or fatigue. With the eyes closed it is impossible to concentrate on the memory or the imagination of a small part of one letter continuously without a temporary or more complete loss of the memory or the imagination.

When an effort is made to think of one part of a letter continuously with the eyes closed, the letter is imagined to be stationary. When the imagination shifts to the right of the letter a short distance and then to the left alternately, every time the attention is directed to the right, the letter is always to the left, and when the attention is directed to the left of the letter, the letter is always to the right. By alternating, the patient becomes able to imagine the letter is moving from side to side, and as long as the movement is maintained the patient is able to remember or imagine the letter. It can be demonstrated that to remember a letter or other object to be stationary always interferes with the perfect memory of the letter. One cannot remember, imagine, or see an object continuously unless it is moving. The movement must be slow, short, and easy.

When patients stare habitually, the eyes become more or less fixed, and are moved with great difficulty. When the patient stands and sways the whole body from side to side, it becomes easier to move the eyes in the same direction as the body moves. No matter how long the staring has been practiced, the sway at once lessens it.

SWAYING

Demonstrate

1. That the sway improves the vision because it prevents the stare.

Stand with the feet about one foot apart, facing a Snellen test card about fifteen feet away. Sway the body from side to side, at first with a rapid, wide swing. When the body, head and eyes sway to the right, observe that the Snellen test card is to the left of where you are looking. Then sway the body, head and eyes to the left. The test card is now to the right of where you are looking. Practice this sway for a few minutes and, without looking at the Snellen test card directly, observe that the whiteness of the card becomes whiter and the black spots on the card become a darker shade of black. The test card appears to move in the direction opposite to the movement of the eyes, while objects beyond the card may move in the same direction as the eyes move.

2. That when the forefinger of one hand is held about six inches in front and to one side of the face, the finger appears to move from side to side in the direction opposite to the movement of the head and eyes.

Close the eyes and let the hand rest in the lap and remember the swing of the finger. Imagine that the hand, which is fastened to the finger, moves with it. Realize that when the hand moves, the wrist, the arm, the elbow and other parts of the body, being joined together, all move with the finger. Now try to imagine the elbow is stationary, while the finger is moving. It is impossible to do this. When the finger moves, you can imagine not only your body, but also the chair on which you are sitting, the floor on which the chair rests, the walls of the room, the whole building with its foundation, in fact, the universe to be moving with the finger. This is called the universal swing and is possible only when the memory, imagination, or the sight is good.

64

Demonstrate

1. That a short, swaying movement improves the vision more than a long sway.

Place the test card at a distance where only the large letter at the top of the card can be distinguished. This may be ten feet, further or nearer. Stand with the feet about one foot apart and sway the body from side to side. When the body sways to the right, look to the right of the card. When the body sways to the left, look to the left of the card. Do not look at the Snellen test card. Sway the body from side to side and look to the right of the Snellen test card, and alternately to the left of it. Note that the test card appears to be moving. Increase the length of the sway and notice that the test card seams to move a longer distance from side to side. Observe the whiteness of the card and the blackness of the letters. Now shorten the sway, which, of course, shortens the movement of the card. The card appears whiter and the letters blacker when the movement of the card is short, than when the movement of the card is long.

2. Demonstrate that when the eyes are stationary, they are under a tremendous strain.

Stand before the Snellen test card at a distance of fifteen or twenty feet. Look directly at one small area of a large letter, which can be seen clearly. Stare at that part of the letter without closing the eyes and without shifting the eyes to some other point. The vision becomes worse and the letter blurs. Stare continuously, and note that the longer you stare, the more difficult it is to keep the eyes focused on that one point or part of the letter. Not only does the stare become more difficult, but the eyes become tired; and by making a greater effort, the eyes pain, or a headache is produced. The stare can cause fatigue of the whole body when the effort is sufficiently strong and prolonged.

16. SWINGING

The Swinging Cure

If you see a letter perfectly, you may note that it appears to pulsate, or move slightly in various directions. If your sight is imperfect, the letter will appear to be stationary. The apparent movement is caused by the unconscious shifting of the eye. The lack of movement is due to the fact that the eye stares, or looks too long at one point. This is an invariable symptom of imperfect sight, and may often be relieved by the following method:

Close your eyes and cover them with the palms of the hands so as to exclude all the light, and shift mentally from one side of a black letter to the other. As you do this, the mental picture of the letter will appear to move back and forth in a direction contrary to the imagined movement of the eye. Just so long as you imagine that the letter is moving, or swinging, you will find that you are able to remember it, and the shorter and more regular the swing, the blacker and more distinct the letter will appear. If you are able to imagine the letter stationary, which may be difficult, you will find that your memory of it will be much less perfect.

Now open your eyes and look first at one side and then at the other of the real letter. If it appears to move in a direction opposite to the movement of the eye, you will find that your vision has improved. If you can imagine the swing of the letter as well with your eyes open as with your eyes closed, as short, as regular and as continuous, your vision will be normal.

Demonstrate

That the long swing not only improves the vision, but also relieves or cures pain, discomfort and fatigue. Stand with the feet about one foot apart, facing squarely one side of the room. Lift the left heel a short distance from the floor while turning the shoulders, head, and eyes to the right, until the line of the shoulders is parallel with the wall. Now turn the body to the left after placing the left heel upon the floor and raising the right heel. Alternate looking from the right wall to the left wall, being careful to move the head and eyes with the movement of the shoulders. When practiced easily, continuously, without effort and without paying any attention to moving objects, one soon becomes conscious that the long swing relaxes the tension of the muscles and nerves.

Stationary objects move with varying degrees of rapidity. Objects located almost directly in front of you appear to move with express train speed and should be very much blurred. It is very important to make no attempt to see clearly objects which seem to be moving very rapidly.

The long swing seems to help patients who suffer from eyestrain during sleep. By practicing the long swing fifty times or more just before retiring and just after rising in the morning, eyestrain during sleep has been prevented or relieved.

It is remarkable how quickly the long swing relieves or prevents pain. I know of no other procedure which can compare with it. The long swing has relieved the pain of facial neuralgia after operative measures had failed. Some patients who have suffered from continuous pain in various parts of the body have been relieved by the long swing, at first temporarily, but by repetition the relief has become more permanent. Hay fever, asthma, seasickness, palpitation of the heart, coughs, acute and chronic colds are all promptly cured by the long swing.

SWINGING

The Variable Swing

Recently I have been impressed very much by the value of the variable swing. By the variable swing is meant the ability to imagine a near object with a longer swing then one more distant. For example, a patient came to me with conical cornea, which is usually considered incurable. I placed a chair five feet away from her eyes, clearly on a line with the Snellen test card located 15 feet distant. When she looked at the Snellen test card and imagined the letters moving an inch or less she could imagine the chair that she was not looking at moving quite a distance.

As is well known the shorter the swing the better the sight. Some persons with unusually good vision have a swing so short that they do not readily recognize it. This patient was able to imagine the chair moving an inch or less and the card on the wall moving a shorter distance. She became able to imagine the chair moving a quarter of an inch and the movement of the Snellen test card at 15 feet was so short that she could not notice it. In the beginning her vision with glasses was poor and without glasses was double, and even the larger letters on the Snellen test card were very much blurred.

Now, when she imagined the chair moving a quarter of an inch and the Snellen test card moving so short a distance that she could not recognize it, the conical cornea disappeared from both eyes and her vision became normal. To me it was one of the most remarkable things I have seen in years. I know of no other treatment that has ever brought about so great a benefit in so bad a case.

The variable swing is something that most people can learn how to practice at their first visit. Some people can do it better than others. The improvement depends directly upon their skill in practicing the variable swing.

The Short Swing

Many people with normal sight can demonstrate the short swing readily. They can demonstrate that with normal vision each small letter regarded moves from side to side about a quarter of an inch or less. By an effort they can stop this short swing, and when they are able to demonstrate that, the vision becomes imperfect almost immediately. Practicing the long swing brings a measure of relaxation and makes it possible for those with imperfect sight to see things moving with a shorter swing. It is a good thing to have the help of someone who can practice the short swing successfully. Ask some friend who has perfect sight without glasses in each eye to practice the variable swing as just described, which is a help to those with imperfect sight who have difficulty in demonstrating the short swing.

Nearsighted patients usually can demonstrate that when the vision is perfect, the diamond type at the reading distance, one letter regarded is seen continuously with a slow, short, easy swing not wider than the diameter of the letter. By staring the swing stops and the vision becomes imperfect. It is more difficult for a nearsighted person to stop the swing of the fine print, letter O, than it is to let it swing. When the sight is very imperfect, it is impossible to obtain the short swing. Many people have difficulty in maintaining mental pictures of any letter or any object. They cannot demonstrate the short swing with their eyes closed until they become able to imagine mental pictures.

The Elliptical Swing

The normal eye when it has normal sight is always able to imagine stationary objects to be moving from side to side about one quarter of an inch, slowly and without effort. This is called the swing. In order that the swing may be continuous, the movement of the head and eyes should be in the orbit of an ellipse, or in an elongated circular direction.

A patient, aged seventy-seven, with beginning cataract in both eyes had a vision of 3/200 when she looked to one side of the card. When she looked directly at the card or the letters, she complained that she could not see them so well, or at all. She was recommended to practice swaying the body from side to side. Every time she moved to the right or to the left, she stopped at the end of the movement and stared, and that prevented relaxation. With the help of the Elliptical Swing, she obtained at once very marked benefit. Her vision was improved almost immediately when she looked directly at the letters, and her vision became worse when she looked to one side of the card.

A young man, aged sixteen, was treated for progressive myopia for a year or longer. His vision improved for a time, then improvement stopped. Some months later his vision had not become permanently improved. Palming and swinging no longer helped him. I noticed that when he would move his head from side to side, he stopped at the end of the swing and stared. When he practiced the Elliptical Swing, his head and eyes moved continuously, and the staring was prevented. At once there was a decided improvement in his vision, and this improvement continued without any relapse.

Demonstrate

1. That perfect sight is not possible unless one imagines a letter to be moving, and that an effort to imagine a letter stationary always fails.

Close your eyes and remember a small letter of the Snellen test card. Imagine that some one is moving the test card a short distance from side to side so that all the letters on the card appear to be moving with the movement of the card. Remember the small letter moving. You can remember it provided you imagine it is moving. Now try to stop this movement by staring at one part of the small letter and imagining that it is stationary. The letter soon becomes blurred.

2. That the circular swing prevents the stare and relieves pain and fatigue.

Hold the forefinger of one hand about six inches in front of one eye and a few inches to the outer side of the face. By moving the head and eyes in a circular or an elliptical orbit, notice that the finger appears to move in the direction opposite to the movement of the head and eyes. Now realize that the hand must move with the finger because the hand and finger are fastened together. When one moves, the other moves in the same direction, up, down, to the right or left. The same fact is true of the arm fastened to the wrist. When the finger moves, the hand, wrist and arm in turn, all move and in the same direction. Likewise when the finger moves, the shoulder moves with it and other parts of the body fastened directly or indirectly to the finger. You may soon become able to imagine the chair on which you are sitting to be fastened indirectly to the finger. When one moves, the other always moves in the same direction. When you become able to imagine all things, one at a time to be moving with the finger, i.e., the universal swing, the stare is prevented and pain and fatigue disappear. The memory, imagination and vision are also improved.

SWINGING

Demonstrate

1. That the drifting swing improves the sight. Take a record of your best vision of the Snellen test card with both eyes together and each eye separately without glasses. Now close your eyes and imagine that you are occupying a canoe which is floating down some creek, river or stream. Imagine that the trees, houses and other stationary objects on either side are moving in the direction opposite to the way in which you are moving.

Another way in which to practice the drifting swing is as follows: With the eyes closed, recall a number of familiar objects which can be remembered easily. Sometimes in the course of a few minutes, fifty or one hundred objects may be remembered quickly and then forgotten. Remember each mental picture by central fixation; that is, think of only one part at a time of the object that you are remembering. Just let your mind drift easily from one object to another, without making any effort. Do not try to hold each object as remembered; forget it quickly. Notice that after practicing the above methods for a few minutes the vision for the test card is improved.

2. That the long swing improves the sight, relieves pain, fatigue and many other nervous symptoms.

Take a record of your best vision of the Snellen test card with both eyes together and each eye separately without glasses. Stand, with the feet about one foot apart, facing a blank wall. Turn the body to the left, at the same time raising the heel of the right foot. Now place the heel of the right foot on the floor in its usual position; then turn the body to the right, lifting the heel of the left foot.

The head and eyes move with the body; do not make any effort to see more distinctly stationary objects which are apparently moving. Practice this fifty to one hundred times, easily, without making any effort. Notice that after practicing, the vision for the test card improves.

The Memory Swing

The memory swing relieves strain and tension as do the long or the short swings which have been described at various times. It is done with the eyes closed while one imagines himself to be looking first over the right shoulder and then over the left shoulder, while the head is moved from side to side. The eyeballs may be seen through the closed eyelids to move from side to side in the same direction as the head is moved. When done properly, the memory swing is just as efficient as the swing which is practiced with the eyes open, whether it be short or long.

The memory swing can be shortened by remembering the swing of a small letter, a quarter of an inch or less, when the eyes are closed.

The memory swing has given relief in many cases of imperfect sight from myopia, astigmatism, and inflammations of the outside of the eyeball as well as inflammations of the inside of the eyeball. It is much easier than the swing practiced with the eyes open and secures a greater amount of relaxation or rest than any other swing. It may be practiced incorrectly, just as any swing may be done wrong, and then no benefit will be obtained.

SWINGING

The Baby Swing

Young babies suffer very much from eyestrain. The tension of the eye muscles is always associated with the tension of all the other muscles of the body. Their restlessness can be explained by this tension. I was talking with an Italian mother in the clinic one day about restless children, and asked her why it was that her baby was always so quiet and comfortable when she came to the clinic, while many other babies at the same time were very restless and unhappy.

"Oh," she said, "I love my baby. I like to hold her in my arms and rock her until she smiles."

"Yes, I know," I said, "but that mother over there is rocking her baby in her arms, and the child is screaming its head off."

"Yes," exclaimed the Italian mother, "but see how she rocks it."

Then I noticed that the other mother threw the child from side to side in a horizontal direction with a rapid, jerky, irregular motion, and the more she jerked the child from side to side, the more restless did it become.

"Now, doctor," said the Italian mother, "you watch me."

I did watch her. Instead of throwing the child rapidly, irregularly, intermittently from side to side, she handled her baby as though it had much value in her eyes, and moved her not in straight lines from side to side, but continuously in slow, short, easy curves. The Italian mother picked up the other mother's child, and soon quieted it by the same swing.

I learned something that day.

Demonstrate

That the optical swing always improves the vision.

Stand before an open window with the feet about one foot apart. Sway the whole body, including the head and eyes, from side to side. When the body moves to the right, the head and eyes also move to the right, while, at the same time, the window and other stationary objects are to the left of where you are looking. When the body sways to the left, the window and other stationary objects are to the right. Be sure that the head and eyes are moving from side to side with the whole body, slowly, without an effort to see.

When the swaying is done rapidly, it is possible to imagine stationary objects are moving rapidly in the opposite direction. While the swinging is being practiced, notice that the window and other stationary objects which are nearer, appear to move in the opposite direction to the movement of the body, head and eyes. Objects beyond the window may appear to move in the same direction as the body, head, and eyes move.

Note that when the body is swaying rapidly, the window and other objects are not seen very clearly; but when the swaying is slowed down and short-ened, so that parts of the window move one-quarter of an inch or less, the vision is improved for those parts of the window regarded. More distant objects, which move in the same direction as the movement of the body, head, and eyes, are also improved with the slow, short, easy swing.

After you have become able to imagine the window to be moving, practice on other objects. All day long, the head and eyes are moving. Notice that stationary objects are moving in the opposite direction to the movement of the head and eyes. To see stationary objects apparently stationary, is a strain which lowers the vision and may cause pain, fatigue, and other discomforts.

SWINGING

The Optimum Swing

The optimum swing is the swing which gives the best results under different conditions.

Most readers of this magazine and of "Perfect Sight Without Glasses" know about the swing. The swing may be spontaneous; that is to say, when one remembers a letter perfectly or sees a letter perfectly and continuously without any volition on his part he is able to imagine that it is a slow, short, easy swing. The speed is about as fast as one would count orally. The width of the swing is not more than the width of the letter, and it is remembered or imagined as easily as it is possible to imagine anything without any effort whatsoever. The normal swing of normal sight brings the greatest amount of relaxation and should be imagined. When one is able to succeed then it becomes the optimum swing under favorable conditions.

Nearsighted persons have this normal optimum swing usually at the near point when the vision is perfect. At the distance where the vision is imperfect the optimum swing is something else. It is not spontaneous but has to be produced by a conscious movement of the eyes and head from side to side and is usually wider than the width of the letter, faster than the normal swing, and not so easily produced.

When one has a headache or a pain in the eyes or in any part of the body the optimum swing is always wider and more difficult to imagine than when one has less strain of the eyes. Under unfavorable conditions the long swing is the optimum swing, but under favorable conditions when the sight is good, the normal swing of the normal eye with normal sight is the optimum swing. The long swing brings a measure of relief when done right and makes it possible to shorten it down to the normal swing of the normal eye.

17. THUMB MOVEMENT

The Thumb Movement

Rest the hand against an immovable surface. Place the ball of the thumb lightly in contact with the forefinger. Now move the end of the thumb in a circle of about one-quarter of an inch in diameter. When the thumb moves in one direction, the forefinger should appear to move in the opposite direction, although in reality it is stationary. In the practice of the universal swing, everything is imagined to be moving in the same direction, except the eyes. With the aid of the thumb movement, however, one can imagine the spine and the head moving opposite to the direction of motion of the thumb, while the eyes, being fastened to the head, also move with the head and hand.

While watching the movement of the thumb, remember imperfect sight. At once, the thumb movement becomes irregular or may stop altogether. Demonstrate that any effort, no matter how slight, to see, remember or imagine, interferes with the movement of the thumb. The thumb is so sensitive to an effort or strain that the slightest effort is at once recorded by the motion.

While watching the movement of the thumb, remember perfect sight. Notice that the movement of the thumb is slow, short, continuous, and restful—with relaxation of all parts of the body.

Many patients have been successfully treated for pain, fatigue, and dizziness with the help of the thumb movement, after other treatment had failed. Some patients with severe pain complain that when they forget to practice the movement of the thumb, the pain comes back.

Not only have patients suffering from pain and symptoms of fatigue been relieved, but an equal number have been relieved of imperfect sight by the correct practice of the thumb movement.

The Sense Of Touch An Aid To Vision

Just as Montessori has found that impressions gained through the sense of touch are very useful in teaching children to read and write, persons with defective sight have found them useful in educating their memory and imagination.

One patient whose visual memory was very imperfect found that if she traced an imaginary black letter on the ball of her thumb with her forefinger, she could follow the imaginary lines with her mind as they were being formed and retain a picture of the letter better than when she gained the impression of it through the sense of sight.

Another patient discovered that when he lost the swing he could get it again by sliding his forefinger back and forth over the ball of his thumb. When he moved his fingers it seemed as if his whole body were moving.

Both these expedients have the advantage of being inconspicuous, and can, therefore, be used anywhere.

The vision was improved in both cases.

Aids To Swinging

It is possible for most people to do a very simple thing—to move the finger nail of the thumb from side to side against the finger nail of one finger. This may be done when the patient is in bed or when up and walking around, in the house, in the street or in the presence of other people, and all without attracting attention. With the aid of the movement of the thumb nail which can be felt and its speed regulated one can at the same time regulate the speed of the short swing.

The length of the swing can also be regulated because it can be demonstrated that when the body moves a quarter of an inch from side to side that one can move the thumb from side to side. If the long swing is too rapid it can be slowed down with the aid of the thumb nail; when it is too long it can be shortened. At times the short swing may become irregular and then it can be controlled by the movement of the thumb nail.

It is very interesting to demonstrate how the short swing is always similar to the movements of the fingernail. One great advantage connected with the short swing is that after a period of time of longer or shorter duration, the swing may stop or it may lengthen. It has been found that the movement of the thumb maintains the short swing of the body, the short swing of the letters or the short swing of any objects which may be seen, remembered or imagined. A letter O with a white center can only be remembered continuously with the eyes closed when it has a slow, short, continuous, regular swing and all without any effort or strain. The imagination may fail at times but the movement of the thumb can be maintained for an indefinite period after a little practice. One can more readily control the movement of the thumb instead of the eye.

18. BREATHING

Breathing

Many patients with imperfect sight are benefited by breathing. One of the best methods is to separate the teeth while keeping the lips closed, breathe deeply as though one were yawning. When done properly one can feel the air cold as it passes through the nose and down the throat. This method of breathing secures a great amount of relaxation of the nose, throat, the body generally including the eyes and ears.

A man aged sixty-five, had imperfect sight for distance and was unable to read fine print without the aid of strong glasses. After practicing deep breathing in the manner described he became able at once to read diamond type quite perfectly, as close as six inches from the eyes. The benefit was temporary but by repetition the improvement became more permanent.

At one time I experimented with a number of patients, first having them hold their breath and test their vision, which was usually lower when they did not breathe. They became able to demonstrate that holding their breath was a strain and caused imperfect sight, double vision, dizziness and fatigue, while the deep breathing at once gave them relief.

There is a wrong way of breathing in which when the air is drawn into the lungs the nostrils contract. This is quite conspicuous among many cases of tuberculosis.

Some teachers of physical culture in their classes while encouraging deep breathing close their nostrils when drawing in a long breath. This is wrong because it produces a strain and imperfect sight. By consciously doing the wrong thing, breathing with a strain, one becomes better able to practice the right way and obtain relaxation and better sight.

Through the habit of frequently practicing deep breathing one obtains a more permanent relaxation of the eyes with more constant good vision.

The Rabbit's Throat

During the past ten years a method of breathing has been practiced which has improved the vision of many patients after other methods had failed. It consists of depressing the lower jaw with the lips closed and lowering the tongue and muscles below the chin. At the same time one breathes in through the nose and throat in a manner somewhat similar to snoring and when done properly one can feel a coolness of the air while it passes down into the lungs.

This method of breathing is accompanied with the eyelids being more widely open in a natural way without staring. The ear passages, nose, and throat dilate. The tube which goes from the throat to the middle ear becomes more widely open, with improved hearing in chronic deafness which does not respond to any other treatment. If one rests the chin with the thumb below it and the forefinger just below the lower lip, one can feel with the thumb the hardening of the muscles below the jaw accompanied with a decided swelling. By practice, the swelling and hardness increase. This suggested the title of the Rabbit's Throat because of a similar swelling below the rabbit's chin. The tension of the other muscles of the body becomes relaxed. There is a wonderful increase of muscular control.

Music teachers have told me that the singing voice becomes much better because of the relaxation of the muscles of the throat. The involuntary muscles of the digestive tract become relaxed in a striking manner with the relief of many symptoms of discomfort. Redness and inflammation of the mucous membranes of the eye, ear, nose and throat and the rest of the body are relieved in a few minutes with the aid of the Rabbit's Throat

19. FUNDAMENTALS

Fundamentals

1. Glasses discarded permanently.

2. Favorable conditions: Light may be bright or dim. The distance of the print from the eyes, where seen best, also varies with people.

3. Central Fixation is seeing best where you are looking.

4. Shifting: With normal sight the eyes are moving all the time. This should be practiced continuously and consciously.

5. Swinging: When the eyes move slowly or rapidly from side to side, stationary objects appear to move in the opposite direction.

6. Long Swing: Stand with the feet about one foot apart, turn the body to the right—at the same time lifting the heel of the left foot. Do not move the head or eyes or pay any attention to the apparent movement of stationary objects. Now place the left heel on the floor, turn the body to the left, raising the heel of the right foot. Alternate. This exercise can be practiced just before retiring at night fifty times or more. When done properly, it is a great rest and relieves pain, fatigue, and other symptoms of imperfect sight.

7. Stationary Objects Moving: By moving the head and eyes a short distance from side to side, one can imagine stationary objects to be moving. Since the normal eye is moving all the time, one should imagine all stationary objects to be moving. Never imagine that you see a stationary object stationary.

8. Palming: The closed eyes may be covered with the palm of one or both hands. The patient should rest the eyes and think of something else that is pleasant.

9. Blinking: The normal eye blinks, or closes and opens very frequently. If one does not blink, the vision always becomes worse.

How To Demonstrate The Fundamental Principle Of Treatment

The object of all the methods used in the treatment of imperfect sight without glasses is to secure rest or relaxation, of the mind first and then of the eyes. Rest always improves the vision. Effort always lowers it. Persons who wish to improve their vision should begin by demonstrating these facts.

Close the eyes and keep them closed for fifteen minutes. Think of nothing particular, or think of something pleasant. When the eyes are opened, it will usually be found that the vision has improved temporarily. If it has not, it will be because, while the eyes were closed, the mind was not at rest.

One symptom of strain is a twitching of the eyelids which can be seen by an observer and felt by the patient with the fingers. This can usually be corrected if the period of rest is long enough.

Many persons fail to secure a temporary improvement of vision by closing their eyes, because they do not keep them closed long enough. Children will seldom do this unless a grown person stands by and encourages them. Many adults also require supervision.

To demonstrate that strain lowers the vision, think of something disagreeable— some physical discomfort, or something seen imperfectly. When the eyes are opened, it will be found that the vision has been lowered. Also stare at one part of a letter on the test card, or try to see the whole letter all alike at one time. This invariably lowers the vision, and may cause the letters to disappear.

Suggestions

1. Imagine things are moving all the time.

When riding in a railroad train, when one looks out of the car window, telegraph poles and other objects, although they are stationary, appear to be moving. To stop the movement is impossible, and the effort to do so may be very uncomfortable. The greater the effort, the greater the discomfort, and is the cause of heart sickness, headaches and nausea. It can be demonstrated that any movement of the head and eyes produces an apparent movement of stationary objects.

2. Blink often.

By blinking is meant, closing and opening both eyes rapidly. When done properly, things are seen continuously and they always move with a quick jump in various directions. Regarding stationary objects without blinking is an effort, a strain which always lowers the vision.

3. Read the Snellen Test Card at fifteen feet as well as you can, every night and morning.

School children and others are often cured of imperfect sight by reading a familiar card, first with both eyes and then with each eye separately. It is the only method practiced which prevents myopia in school children.

4. Fine Print.

Read fine print at six inches when possible every night and morning. If not possible, do the best you can. Just regarding the white spaces between the lines of fine print without reading the letters is a benefit.

5. Palming,

Palm for five minutes, ten times daily when convenient.

Improve Your Sight

When convenient, practice the long swing. Stand with the feet about one foot apart, turn the body to the right, at the same time lifting the heel of the left foot. The head and eyes move with the body. Now place the left heel on the floor, turn the body to the left, raising the heel of the right foot. Alternate.

Rest your eyes continually by blinking. The normal eye blinks irregularly but continuously. When convenient, practice blinking in the following way: Count irregularly and blink for each count. By consciously blinking correctly, it will in time become an unconscious habit.

When the mind is awake it is thinking of many things. One can remember things perfectly or imagine things perfectly, which is a rest to the eyes, mind, and the body generally. The memory of imperfect sight should be avoided because it is a strain and lowers the vision.

Read the Snellen test card at 20 feet with each eye, separately, twice daily or oftener when convenient. Imagine the white spaces in letters to be whiter than the rest of the card. Do this alternately with the eyes closed and opened. Plan to imagine the white spaces in letters just as white, in looking at the Snellen test card, as can be accomplished with the eyes closed.

Whenever convenient, close your eyes for a few minutes and rest them.

Demonstrate

1. That a strain to see at the distance produces nearsightedness. Look at a Snellen test card at twenty feet and read it as well as you can. Now strain or make an effort to see it better, and note that instead of becoming better, it becomes worse.

2. That a strain to see at the near point does not increase nearsightedness, but always lessens it.

Look at a card of fine print at six inches from your eyes and read it as well as you can. Now make an effort to see it better, and note that your vision for the near point is lowered, while the ability to read the fine print at a greater distance is improved.

3. That when a mental picture is perfect with the eyes closed for part of a minute or longer, a perfect mental picture can be remembered, imagined, or seen for a second or less with the eyes open.

Remember a black kitten. If your mental picture is gray or an imperfect black with the eyes closed, imagine that you are pouring black ink or black dye over it. Note that the clearness of the mental picture improves.

Look at a page of fine print. Then close your eyes and imagine the white spaces between the lines to be perfectly white. If they appear to be a grayish white, imagine that you are painting the white spaces between the letters, inside the letters, and between the lines, with white paint or whitewash. Then open your eyes for a fraction of a second and note that the white spaces between the lines will appear whiter, if you do not make an effort to see either the black letters or the white spaces.

Demonstrate

1. That an effort to see always lowers the vision. Look at the Snellen test card at a distance of twenty feet. It may be possible for you to see the large letters and read them without any apparent effort, while the smaller letters produce a strain which you can feel. If you consciously increase the effort to see the smaller letters, your vision becomes more imperfect. It is not easy for you to realize that effort is always present when the vision is lowered. Knowing the cause of your imperfect sight is a great help in selecting the remedy.

2. That a stare always lowers the vision. It is a truth that the normal eye blinks very frequently. In order to have normal sight, the eyes must blink. One can demonstrate that, when the patient looks at one letter at the distance with normal sight, or looks at one letter at a near point where it is seen clearly, keeping the eyes continuously open without blinking for a minute or longer, always lowers the vision for the distance or for the near point. This should convince the patient that blinking is absolutely necessary in order to obtain good vision.

3. That palming, when done correctly, improves the vision. When the closed eyes are covered with one or both hands, and all light is excluded, the patient should see nothing at all, or a perfect black. This is a rest to the eyes and always improves the sight at least temporarily. Palming can be done wrong. When it is practiced incorrectly, the field imagined by the patient contains streaks of red, white, blue, or other colors. The eyes are under a strain, and the vision is not materially improved by the wrong method of palming. It can be demonstrated that palming for half an hour or longer is a greater benefit than palming for only a few minutes.

The Trinity

There are three things which the normal eye practices more or less continuously, which are necessary in order to maintain normal vision.

1—The long swing.

2—The short swing.

3—Blinking or palming.

The long swing has been described repeatedly and most people are able to practice it successfully, especially people whose sight is good. If you have very imperfect sight you may have difficulty in demonstrating the benefit of the long swing. Some patients are indeed difficult to manage. They may be able to practice the long swing when looking out of a window with its light background. By moving the whole body, head and eyes together, a long distance from side to side one becomes able to imagine a cord of the window shade moving in the opposite direction. This makes it possible to imagine the long swing when you turn your back to the window, and look at objects in the room which have a dark background.

When the long swing is properly maintained the letters of the Snellen Test Card become darker as long as one does not look directly at the card. Looking above the card or below it is a help in maintaining the long swing of the card when the maximum vision is obtained by the long swing. Never look directly at the card or try to read the letters when practicing the long swing.

By gradually lessening the movement of the body from side to side, the swing of the card becomes shorter and one may soon become able to flash the large letters. The swing of the card can be reduced to an inch or less.

One Thing

By CENTRAL FIXATION is meant the ability to see one letter or one object regarded in such a way that all other letters or objects are seen worse. Some people have been cured by practicing Central Fixation only, devoting little time to other methods of cure.

SWINGING

When the normal eye has normal sight the small letters of the Snellen Test Card are imagined to be moving from side to side, slow, continuously, not more than the width of the letter. Persons with imperfect sight have become able to imagine this illusion by alternately remembering or imagining the small letter moving from side to side continuously. With their eyes open they may be able to do it for a moment or flash it, at first occasionally, and later more continuously, until they are cured.

IMAGINATION is very efficient in improving the vision. Some persons have told me that when they knew what a letter was they could imagine they saw it. By closing their eyes they usually became able to imagine a known letter better than with their eyes open. By alternately imagining a known letter with the eyes open and with the eyes closed, the imagination of the letter often improves to normal when the letter was regarded. The patient who is able to do this is also able to demonstrate that when the imagination is improved for one known letter the vision for unknown letters is also improved. By imagining the first letter of a line perfectly the patient can tell the second letter and other letters which are not known. The imagination cure is curative when other methods of treatment have failed.

20. PRACTICING

Practicing

A great many people have asked, "How much time should one devote to practicing the methods of central fixation in order to be cured of imperfect sight without glasses?"

The answer is—ALL THE TIME.

One should secure relaxation or rest until one is perfectly comfortable and continue feeling comfortable as long as one is awake.

The feeling of relaxation or comfort can be obtained with the memory of perfect sight. Even if one cannot remember perfect sight one can imagine it. All black objects should be imagined perfectly black. All white objects observed should be imagined perfectly white. All letters observed should be imagined perfectly and everything that is seen should be imagined perfectly.

To imagine anything imperfectly requires a strain, an effort, which is difficult. Choose the easy way. Imagine things perfectly.

If you try to imagine an object as stationary you will strain and your sight become impaired. All day long the eyes are moving from one point to another. Imagine that objects are moving opposite to the movement of the eyes. If one does not notice this one is very apt to strain and imagine things stationary.

One can practice properly for ten minutes and be comfortable. That does not mean that all the rest of the day one can strain and tear one's eyes all to pieces without paying the penalty for breaking the law. If you are under treatment for imperfect sight be sure to keep in mind all day long from the time you wake up in the morning until you go to bed at night the feeling of comfort, of rest, of relaxation, incessantly. It is a great deal better to do that than to feel under a strain and be uncomfortable all day long.

Practice Methods

Many people have asked for help in choosing the best method of treatment for their particular eye trouble. A woman aged sixty complained that she had never been free of pain; pain was very decided in her eyes and head. She also had continuous pain in nearly all the nerves of the body. The long swing when practiced 100 times gave her great relief from pain. The relief was continuous without any relapse. At the same time a second woman of about the same age complained of a similar pain which, like the first patient, she had had almost continuously. She was also relieved by practicing the long swing. The long swing was practiced by other people with a satisfactory result.

It seemed that the swing was indicated for pain; it seemed to bring about better results than any other treatment. Later on, however, some patients applied for relief from pain which was not benefited by the long swing. Evidently one kind of treatment was not beneficial in every case. A man suffering from tri-facial neuralgia which caused great agony in all parts of the head was not relieved at all by the long swing. Palming seemed to be more successful in bringing about relief. Furthermore, there were patients who did not obtain benefit after half an hour of palming who did obtain complete relief after palming for several hours.

Patients with cataract recovered quite promptly when some special method was tried.

The experience obtained by the use of relaxation methods in the cure of obstinate eye troubles has proved that what was good for one patient was not necessarily a benefit to other patients suffering from the same trouble, and that various methods must be tried in each case in order to determine which is the most beneficial for each particular case.

Time To Practice

Many busy people complain that they have not time to practice my methods. They say that wearing glasses is quicker and much easier. Persons with normal vision or perfect sight without glasses are practicing consciously or unconsciously all the time when they are awake. When one sees a letter or an object perfectly the eyes are at rest. Any effort to improve the sight always makes it worse. The only time the eyes are perfectly at rest is when the vision is perfect. Persons with imperfect sight have to strain in order to see imperfectly. Persons with headaches, pain and other symptoms of discomfort in the eyes or in other parts of the body are under a constant strain to see, which is usually unconscious.

When a patient says he has no time to practice he is mistaken. He has all the time there is to use his eyes in the right way, or he can use them in the wrong way. He has just as much time to use his eyes properly as he has to use them improperly. He has the choice and when patients learn the facts, to complain that they have no time to practice is an error.

Some patients object to removing their glasses on the ground that their vision is not sufficiently good for them to attend to their work, and feel that they have to put off the treatment until they have a vacation. Some of my patients have very poor vision and yet find time to practice without their glasses. Some school teachers with 15 diopters of myopia with a vision of less than 10/200 have found time to practice without interfering with their work. In fact practicing without their glasses soon enabled them to do their work much better than before.

Time For Practice

So many people with imperfect sight say that they have not the time to practice relaxation methods, as their time is taken up at business or in the performance of other duties. I always tell such people, however, that they have just as much time to use their eyes correctly as incorrectly.

They can imagine stationary objects to be moving opposite whenever they move their head and eyes. When the head and eyes move to the left, stationary objects should appear to move to the right, and vice versa.

They can remember to blink their eyes in the same way that the normal eye blinks unconsciously, which is frequently, rapidly, continuously, without any effort or strain, until by conscious practice, it will eventually become an unconscious habit, and one that will be of benefit to the patient.

They can remember to shift or look from one point to another continuously. When practicing shifting, it is well to move the head in the same direction as the eyes move. If the head moves to the right, the eyes should move to the right. If the head moves to the left, the eyes should move to the left. By practicing in this way, relaxation is often obtained very quickly, but if the eyes are moved to the right and at the same time the head is moved to the left, a strain on the nerves of the eyes and the nerves of the body in general is produced.

PRACTICING

Practice Time

A large number of people have bought the book "Perfect Sight Without Glasses" but do not derive as much benefit from it as they should because they do not know how long they should practice.

Rest: The eyes are rested in various ways. One of the best methods is to close the eyes for half an hour after testing the sight. This usually improves the vision.

Palming: With the eyes closed and covered with the palms of both hands the vision is usually benefited. The patient should do this five minutes hourly.

Shifting: The patient looks from one side of the room to the other, alternately resting the eyes. This may be done three times daily for half an hour at a time. The head should move with the eyes and the patient should blink.

Swinging: When the shifting is slow, stationary objects appear to move from side to side. This should be observed whenever the head and eyes move.

Long Swing: Nearly all persons should practice the long swing one hundred times daily.

Memory: When the vision is perfect, it is impossible for the memory to be imperfect. One can improve the memory by alternately remembering a letter with the eyes open and closed. This should be practiced for half an hour twice daily.

Imagination: It has been frequently demonstrated and published in this magazine that the vision is only what we imagine it to be. Imagination should be practiced whenever the vision is tested. Imagine a known letter with the eyes open and with the eyes closed. This should be practiced for ten minutes twice daily.

Repetition: When one method is found which improves the vision more than any other method, it should be practiced until the vision is continuously improved.

Improve Your Sight

All day long use your eyes right. You have just as much time to use your eyes right as you have to use them wrong. It is easier and more comfortable to have perfect sight than to have imperfect sight.

Practice the long swing. Notice that when your eyes move the great distance rapidly, objects in front of you move in the opposite direction so rapidly that you do not see them clearly. Do not try to see them because that stops the apparent movement.

Rest your eyes continually by blinking, which means to open and close them so rapidly that one appears to see things continuously. Whenever convenient close your eyes for a few minutes and rest them. Cover them with one or both hands to shut out the light and obtain a greater rest.

When the mind is awake it is thinking of many things. One can remember things perfectly or imagine things perfectly, which is a rest to the eyes, mind and the body generally. The memory of imperfect sight should be avoided because it is a strain and lowers the vision.

Read the Snellen Test Card at 20 feet with each eye separately, twice daily or oftener. Imagine white spaces in letters whiter than the rest of the card. Do this alternately with the eyes closed and opened. Plan to imagine the white spaces in letters just as white, in looking at the Snellen test card, as can be accomplished with the eyes closed.

Remember one letter of the alphabet, or a part of one letter, or a period, continuously and perfectly.

Permanent Improvement

Many patients find that while it is easy for them to obtain a temporary improvement in their sight by palming a sufficient length of time or by other methods, they do not seem to hold it permanently. In this connection it is well to remember that the normal eye with normal sight can only maintain normal sight permanently by consciously or unconsciously practicing the slow, short, easy swing. When the normal eye has imperfect sight it can always be demonstrated that the swing stops from an effort.

When the normal eye has normal sight, the eyes are at rest and all the nerves of the body feel comfortable. When the swing stops, one always feels more or less uncomfortable. To have perfect sight can only be obtained easily, without effort. To have imperfect sight always requires a strain or an effort which stops the swing. Nearsighted patients who have normal vision for reading at the near point become able, when their attention is called to it, to demonstrate that they are more comfortable when reading the fine print than they are when they fail to see distant objects perfectly.

One of the great benefits of the drifting swing is the comfortable relaxed feeling it brings. The retinoscope always shows that the eye is not nearsighted when no effort is made. Persons with imperfect sight should imitate the eye with normal sight by practicing a perfect memory, a perfect imagination, a perfect swing, without effort, with perfect comfort all the time that they are awake. As I have said before many times, it is a good thing to know what is the matter with you because it makes it possible to correct it.

Favorable Conditions

The vision of the human eye is modified in many ways when the conditions are unfavorable to good sight. Unfavorable conditions may prevail when the light is not agreeable to the patient. Some patients require a very bright light and others get along much better in a poor light. Many cases are hypersensitive to the light and suffer from an intolerance for light which has been called photophobia.

While intolerance of light may be manifest in most cases from some diseases of the eyes, there are many cases in which the eye is apparently healthy and in which the photophobia may be extreme. (The cure for this condition is to have the patient sit in the sun with his eyes closed, allowing the sun to shine on his closed eyelids as he moves his head from side to side.)

There are patients with good sight whose vision is materially improved when used in a bright light, as well as those with good sight whose vision improves when the eyes are used in a dim light. The patient should practice with the test card in a bright as well as a dim light to accustom his eyes to all conditions.

The ability to perceive halos, or an increased whiteness, around letters is a favorable condition. By using a screen or a fenestrated card, it is possible for many patients to see an increased whiteness around a letter, which improves their vision for the letter. When a screen is not used, one may be able to imagine a white halo around the inner or outer edge of the black part of the "O." When a screen covers the black part of the letter "O" for instance, the white center becomes of the same whiteness as the rest of the white page, which proves that it is the contrast between the black and the white which enables one to imagine the white halos. The presence of the black improves the white; the presence of the white improves the black.

21. CHILDREN

Children May Improve Their Sight By Consciously Doing The Wrong Thing

Children often make a great effort to see the blackboard and other distant objects in school. It helps them to overcome this habit to have them demonstrate just what the strain to see does.

Tell them to fix their attention on the smallest letter they can see from their seats, to stare at it, to concentrate on it, to partly close their eyelids—in short, to make as great an effort as possible to see it.

The letter will blur, or disappear altogether, and the whole card may become blurred, while discomfort, or pain in the eyes or head, will be produced.

Now direct them to rest their eyes by palming. The pain or discomfort will cease, the letter will come out again, and other letters that they could not see before may come out also.

After a demonstration like this children are less likely to make an effort to see the blackboard, or anything else; but some children have to repeat the experiment many times before the subconscious inclination to strain is corrected.

School Children's Eyes

The cure and prevention of imperfect sight in school children is very simple.

A Snellen Test Card should be placed in the class room where all children can see it from their seats. They should read the card at least once daily with each eye separately, covering the other eye with the palms of the hands, in such a way as to avoid pressing on the eyeball. The time required is less than a minute for both eyes. The card measures the amount of their vision. They will find from time to time that their eyesight varies. Some children are very much disturbed when they cannot see so well on account of the light being dim on a dark or rainy day and although they usually learn the letters by heart they do not always remember or see them. It is well to encourage the children to commit the letters to memory because it is a great help for them to see them. When a child can read the Snellen Test Card with each eye with perfect sight, even although they do know what the letters are, it has been found by numerous observations that their eyes are also normal and not nearsighted, farsighted nor do they have astigmatism. Many children find that when they have difficulty in reading the writing on the blackboard that they obtain material help after glancing at the Snellen Test Card and reading it with perfect sight.

When the eye is at rest, perfect rest, it always has perfect sight. A great many teachers and others condemn the method unwisely because they say that the children learn, and because they know what the letters are, they recite them without actually seeing them. With my instrument I have observed many thousands of school children reading the Snellen Test Card apparently with perfect sight, the test card that they had committed to memory, and in all cases never did I find anything wrong with their eyes.

About ten years ago I challenged a Doctor, a member of the Board of Education, to prove that the children deceive themselves or others by saying that they see letters when they don't. To me it is very interesting that the most wicked child in school no matter how he may lie about other things with great facility and gets by with it, was never caught lying about his eyesight. I believe that every family should have a Snellen Test Card in the home and the children encouraged to practice reading it for a few minutes or longer a number of times every day. Some children are fond of contests and quite often a child who can demonstrate that his vision was the best of any pupil in the class had a feeling of pride and satisfaction which every one in sporting events can understand.

The Cure Of Imperfect Sight In School Children

While reading the Snellen test card every day will, in time, cure imperfect sight in all children under twelve who have never worn glasses, the following simple practices will insure more rapid progress:

1. Let the children rest their eyes by closing for a few minutes or longer, and then look at the test card for a few moments only, then rest again, and so on alternately. This cures many children very promptly.

2. Let them close and cover their eyes with the palms of their hands in such a way as to exclude all the light while avoiding pressure on the eyeballs (palming), and proceed as above. This is usually more effective than mere closing.

3. Let them demonstrate that all effort lowers the vision by looking fixedly at a letter on the test card, or at the near point, and noting that it blurs or disappears in less than a minute. They thus become able, in some way, to avoid unconscious effort.

The method succeeds best when the teachers do not wear glasses.

Supervision is absolutely necessary. At least once a year some person whose sight is normal without glasses and who understands the method should visit the classrooms for the purpose of answering questions, testing the sight of the children, and making a report to the proper authorities.

The Snellen test card is a chart showing letters of graduated sizes, with numbers indicating the distance in feet at which each line should be read by the normal eye. Originally designed by Snellen for the purpose of testing the eye, it is admirably adapted for use in eye education.

The Prevention Of Myopia

The August number of Better Eyesight is a school number devoted almost exclusively to the problem of the cure or prevention of nearsightedness in school children. The great value of the method as a preventive is emphasized by the fact that the vision of all school children has always improved, and when the vision is improved of course imperfect sight is prevented. It is well to remember that my method for the prevention of myopia in school children is the only one that is a success. It has been in continuous use for more than twenty years in the public schools of New York and other cities. Once daily or oftener the children read the card, first with one eye and then with the other, covering each eye alternately with the palm of the hand in such a way as to shut out all the light without any pressure on the eyeball.

Teachers who have studied my book or have been patients find it an advantage to have the children palm five minutes three or four times a day. They claim that palming quiets the children and gives them an improved mental efficiency, which is a great help to their memory and imagination as well as their sight. I believe other children should be taught how to palm, swing, blink and improve their vision of the Snellen Test Card. The method is of great value to young children in the kindergarten, children in the high schools, and should be practiced by students and teachers in colleges and universities. In the military school and naval academy the method should be employed for the prevention of imperfect sight.

22. VARIOUS TOPICS

Methods That Have Succeeded In Presbyopia

The cure of presbyopia, as of any other error of refraction, is rest, and many presbyopic patients are able to obtain this rest simply by closing the eyes. They are kept closed until the patient feels relieved, which may be in a few minutes, half an hour, or longer. Then some fine print is regarded for a few seconds. By alternately resting the eyes and looking at fine print many patients quickly become able to read it at eighteen inches, and by continued practice they are able to reduce the distance until it can be read at six inches in a dim light. At first the letters are seen only in flashes. Then they are seen for a longer time, until finally they are seen continuously. When this method fails, palming may be tried, combined with the use of the memory, imagination and swing. Particularly good results have been obtained from the following procedure:

Close the eyes and remember the letter o in diamond type [ₒ], with the open space as white as starch and the outline as black as possible.

When the white center is at the maximum imagine that the letter is moving, and that all objects, no matter how large or small, are moving with it.

Open the eyes and continue to imagine the universal swing.

Alternate the imagination of the swing with the eyes open with its imagination with the eyes closed.

When the imagination is just as good with the eyes open as when they are closed the cure will be complete.

Floating Specks

When a patient stares or strains to see by looking at a light-colored surface he may see, or imagine he sees, floating black specks, strings of black thread or small light-colored globules resembling tears. The floating specks may be apparently a quarter of an inch or more in size and they may be of any shape.

The ability to see or imagine floating specks may occur in children or in adults of any age. Some children have been known to lie on their backs on the ground, look up at light colored clouds and amuse themselves for hours by watching what appeared to be floating specks.

Many nervous people have been made very unhappy, consciously or unconsciously imagining that they see these floating specks.

The cause of floating specks is an imperfect memory of perfect sight. Persons with normal vision who have never been conscious of floating specks can be taught how to imagine them by straining – to imagine letters, colors or other objects imperfectly.

Conversely, patients who are conscious of floating specks are unable to image them and perfect sight at the same time.

In the treatment of floating specks it is important to convince the patients thoroughly that they are only imagined and not seen. It helps very much to impress on the patient's mind that to see these floating specks requires a sufficient strain to lose a perfect imagination of all objects seen, remembered or imagined at all times and in all places.

Multiple Vision

Persons with imperfect sight when they regard one letter of the Snellen Test Card or one letter of fine print instead of seeing just one letter they may see two, three, six or more letters. Sometimes these letters are arranged side by side, sometimes in a vertical line one above the other and in other cases they may be arranged oblique by any angle. Multiple vision can be produced at will by an effort. It can always be corrected by relaxation. One of the best methods is to close the eyes and cover them in such a way as to exclude the light. Do this for five minutes or a half hour or long enough to obtain normal sight. The double vision is then corrected. Practice of the long swing is a great help.

When the long swing is done properly the multiple images are always lessened. Do not forget that you can do the long swing in the wrong way and increase the multiple images. One great advantage of the long swing is that it helps you to obtain a slow, short, continuous swing of normal sight. When the vision is normal the letters appear to move from side to side or in some other direction a distance of about a quarter of an inch. The speed is about equal to the time of the moving feet of soldiers on the march.

The most important part of the short swing is that it should be maintained easily. Any effort or strain modifies or stops the short swing. Then the eyes begin to stare and the multiple images return. It is a great benefit to learn how to produce multiple images at will because this requires much effort or strain, and is decidedly more difficult than normal single vision which can only be obtained easily without effort.

Make Your Squint Worse

There is no better way of curing squint than by making it worse, or by producing other kinds of squint. This can be done as follows:

To produce convergent squint, strain to see a point about three inches from the eyes, such as the end of the nose. To produce divergent squint, fix a point at the distance to one side of any object, and strain to see it as well as when directly regarded.

To produce a vertical squint, look at a point below an object at the distance, and at the same time strain to see the latter.

To produce an oblique divergent squint, look at a point below and to one side of an object at the distance while straining to see the latter.

When successful two images will be seen arranged horizontally, vertically, or obliquely, according to the direction of the strain.

The production of convergent squint is usually easier than that of the other varieties, and most patients succeed better with a light as the object of vision than with a letter, or other non-luminous object.

The Treatment Of Cataract

From "A Case of Cataract," by Victoria Coolidge, in "Better Eyesight" for June, 1920.

The treatment prescribed was as follows:

Palming six times a day, a half hour or longer at a time.

Reading the Snellen test card at five, ten, and twenty feet.

Reading fine print at six inches, five minutes at a time, especially soon after rising in the morning and just before retiring at night, and reading books and newspapers.

Besides this, he was to subject his eyes, especially the left, to the sunlight whenever an opportunity offered, to drink twelve glasses of water a day, walk five miles a day, and later, when he was in better training, to run half a mile or so every day.

The results of this treatment have been most gratifying. Not only have his eyes improved steadily, but his general health has been so much benefited that at eighty-two he looks, acts and feels better and younger than he did at eighty-one.

Voluntary Production Of Eye Tension A Safeguard Against Glaucoma

It is a good thing to know how to increase the tension of the eyeball voluntarily, as this enables one to avoid not only the strain that produces glaucoma, but other kinds of strain also. To do this proceed as follows:

Put the fingers on the upper part of the eyeball while looking downward, and note its softness. Then do any one of the following things:

Try to see a letter, or other object, imperfectly, or (with the eyes either closed or open) to imagine it imperfectly.

Try to see a letter, or a number of letters, all alike at one time, or to imagine them in this way.

Try to imagine that a letter, or mental picture of a letter, is stationary.

Try to see a letter, or other object, double, or to imagine it double.

When successful the eyeball will become harder in proportion to the degree of the strain; but, as it is very difficult to see, imagine, or remember, things imperfectly, all may not be able at first to demonstrate the facts.

Color Blindness

Some people are unable to distinguish red from blue or other colors. Many doctors explain color blindness to be due to something wrong with the retina, optic nerve or brain. They believe that organic changes in the retina are the principal cause. But this is not always true because, in some cases, cures occur without any apparent change in the retina.

I have found that color blindness occurs in a great many cases in an eye apparently normal. There are, however, a number of individuals who can be demonstrated to have color blindness as a result of a disease of the retina caused by mental strain. These cases cannot be cured, however, until the disease of the retina is cured.

Some patients with color blindness are sensitive to a bright light. On the other hand, there are patients with color blindness who are more comfortable in a bright light. These patients are usually relieved by the practice of sun treatment, central fixation, palming, the long swing, or any other method which brings about relaxation.

One patient had a normal perception for colors at three feet and at ten feet. But at a nearer point than three feet she was color blind, the blindness being most marked at three inches. At a distance greater than ten feet the color blindness was evident. After her eyestrain was relieved by relaxation her color blindness disappeared.

People who have been born color blind as well as those who have acquired color blindness have all been cured by the practice of relaxation methods.

How To Obtain Perception Of Light In Blindness

Two things have always brought perception of light to blind patients. One is palming, and the other is the swing.

The swing may take two forms:

1. Let the patient stand with feet apart, and sway the body, including the head and eyes, from side to side, while shifting the weight from one foot to the other.

2. Let him move his hand from one side to the other in front of his face, all the time trying to imagine that he sees it moving. As soon as he becomes able to do this it can be demonstrated that he really does see the movement.

Simple as these measures are they have always, either singly or together, brought relaxation, and with it perception of light, in from fifteen minutes or less to half an hour.

In palming the patient should remember that this does not bring relief unless mental relaxation is obtained, as evidenced by the disappearance of the white, grey and other colors which most blind people see at first with their eyes closed and covered.

Subjective Conjunctivitis

By subjective conjunctivitis is meant that the conjunctiva is inflamed without the evidence of disease. Many people with subjective conjunctivitis will complain of a foreign body in the eye and yet careful search with the use of a good light and a strong magnifying glass will reveal no foreign body present.

Some people with subjective conjunctivitis complain that they have granulated lids and that they suffer from time to time from the presence of little pimples on the inside of the eyelids and the pain that they suffer is out of proportion to the cause that they give to it. Among the many symptoms of subjective conjunctivitis may be a flow of tears from very slight irritants. However, the tear ducts, with the aid of which the tears are drained from the eye, are usually open in these cases and they are sufficiently open to receive a solution of boracic acid which may be injected through the tear duct into the nose. This shows that the tear duct is open normally, and therefore can drain the tears from the eyes.

Dr. C. R. Agnew, at one time professor of ophthalmology at Columbia University, gave many lectures on subjective conjunctivitis in 1885 and 1886. The treatment which he advocated was dry massage of the whole body and I can testify that it was an excellent remedy. However, the treatment which I found was the greatest benefit was the aqueous extract of the suprarenal capsule, or adrenalin, the properties of which I discovered, using one drop in each eye three times a day.

Many cases were benefited by the sun treatment, by central fixation and by the practice of the universal swing.

Influenza—A Quick Cure

When the muscles of the eyes are perfectly relaxed all errors of refraction are not only corrected, but abnormal conditions in other parts of the body are also relieved. It is impossible to relax the muscles of the eyes without relaxing every other muscle in the body.

When people have colds or influenza the muscles that control the circulation in the affected parts are under a strain, the arteries are contracted, and the heart is not able to force the normal amount of blood through them. The blood consequently accumulates in the veins and produces inflammation. Hence any treatment which relaxes the muscles of the eyes sufficiently to produce central fixation and normal vision will cure colds and influenza.

When one palms perfectly, shifts easily, or has a perfect universal swing, not only the muscles which control the refraction, but the muscles of the arteries which control the circulation of the eyes, nose, lungs, kidneys, etc., are relaxed, and all symptoms of influenza disappear. The nasal discharge ceases as if by magic, the cough is at once relieved, and if the nose has been closed, it opens. Pain, fatigue, fever and chilliness are also relieved. The truth of these statements has been repeatedly demonstrated.

The Editor is very proud of this discovery which is now published for the first time.

The Prevention And Control Of Pain By The Mind

Anyone who has normal vision can demonstrate in a few moments that when the memory is perfect no pain is felt, and can produce pain by an attempt to keep the attention fixed on a point. To do this proceed as follows:

Look at a black letter, close the eyes and remember it. Look at the letter again and again close the eyes and remember it. Repeat until the memory is equal to the sight. Now press the nail of one finger against the tip of another. If the letter is remembered perfectly, no pain will be felt. With practice it may become possible to remember the letter with the eyes open.

Remember the letter imperfectly, with blurred edges and clouded openings, and again press the nail of one finger against the tip of another. In this case it will be found impossible to continue the pressure for more than a moment on account of the pain.

Try to remember one point of a letter continuously. It will be found impossible to do so, and if the effort is continued long enough pain will be produced.

Try to look continuously at one point of a letter or other object. If the effort is continued long enough, pain will be produced.

First Visit Cures

The word "cures" is used advisedly. It is a fact that some people have been cured of myopia in one visit, after relaxation of the nerves of the eyes and other parts of the body was obtained.

Suppose the patient is nearsighted and can only see the big letter "C" at fifteen feet, a vision of 15/200. Let the patient walk up close to the card until he can read the bottom line. The distance may be three feet, five feet, or farther. The first letter on the bottom line may be the letter "F". With the eyes open, it is possible for the patient to imagine "F" quite perfectly, but with the eyes closed, he is more easily able to remember and imagine he sees the letter "F" much better.

Palming is a great help when remembering or imagining the letter "F" with the eyes closed. By alternately imagining the letter "F" with the eyes open, and remembering or imagining it better with the eyes closed, the memory, the imagination and finally the vision for the letter "F" is very much improved.

If the patient becomes able to see the letter "F" at three feet, or to imagine he sees it quite perfectly, he should be encouraged to walk back and increase the distance between the eyes and the letter "F" about one foot. When the patient becomes able to imagine the letter "F" at four feet, he should go back another foot, alternately imagining it with his eyes open and remembering it much better with his eyes closed. By gradually increasing the distance of the eyes from the letter "F," all patients who practiced this method obtained normal vision temporarily at the first visit.

The length of time required to obtain a permanent cure is variable. Some patients with not more than one or two diopters of myopia may require many weeks or months of daily treatment before they are permanently cured, while others with a higher degree of myopia sometimes obtain a cure in a much shorter time.

VARIOUS TOPICS

The Book Perfect Sight Without Glasses

A great many people have testified that they were cured by the help that they obtained from the book. A large number I believe have failed to be cured with its help although most people have been able to get some benefit from it.

On the first page is described the Fundamental Principle. This should interest most people because if you can follow the directions recommended you will most certainly be cured of imperfect sight from various causes. If you have a serious injury to the eye which destroys some of its essential parts you will find it impossible to carry out the directions. At the bottom of the page is printed: "If you fail ask some one with perfect sight to help you."

It is an interesting fact that only people with perfect sight without glasses can demonstrate the Fundamental Principle. You will read that with your eyes closed you should rest them, which is not possible if you remember things imperfectly. The book recommends that you remember some color that you can remember perfectly because it has been demonstrated that the normal eye is always at rest when it has normal sight. A perfect memory means perfect rest. Should you have perfect rest you have perfect sight. Most people can demonstrate that they can remember some letter or other object or some color better with their eyes closed than with their eyes open. By practice some people become able to remember, imagine and see mental pictures as well with their eyes open as they can with their eyes closed. Then they are cured.

Correspondence Treatment

Many letters are received from people in various parts of the world who find it impossible to come to New York and who believe that something might be done for them by correspondence treatment. I do not advocate correspondence treatment as a general rule, as the results are uncertain. There is always the possibility that the patient will not practice correctly the things which he is told to do.

If a patient has had one treatment at my office or at the office of one of my representatives, it is possible to treat that patient more intelligently through correspondence.

Some years ago a gentleman living a thousand miles from New York called and asked if anything could be done through correspondence for his wife who was bedridden and suffering with an agony of pain in her eyes. He described all her symptoms to me and gave me her last prescription for glasses. He was told that if he would take the treatment in my office, and so learn how to treat his wife, it would be possible for him to aid her intelligently when he went home. He did this and after taking several treatments, returned. He wrote me later saying that his wife was almost cured.

When my book, "Perfect Sight Without Glasses," is read carefully, those things which are not understood may be cleared up by intelligent questions, which I am always pleased to answer. I do not consider this as regular correspondence treatment.

Questions

Asking questions is all too common with patients who have imperfect sight. There are important or necessary questions which the patient should know in order to bring about a cure. The cause of the imperfect sight should be emphasized. In all cases of imperfect sight a strain, an effort, a stare or concentration can be demonstrated. To see imperfectly requires a great deal of trouble. Even the imperfect memory or the memory or imagination of an imperfect letter is an effort. It is so great a strain that the memory or imagination fail if you keep it in mind for any length of time. Perfect sight can only be obtained without an effort, without a strain. It is impossible to remember or imagine things perfectly by an effort.

One may divide questions into (1)—Proper questions; (2)—Improper or useless questions. It is a waste of time, an injury to the patient, for him to describe the infinite manifestations of imperfect sight. To know its history minutely and its variations require an effort on the part of the patient to describe these things. And this effort increases the imperfect sight. It is absolutely of no help whatever in formulating methods for its cure. Avoid asking questions about the symptoms of imperfect sight or anything connected with imperfect sight. Any question connected with perfect sight may be a good thing for the patient to know. One may ask questions as follows:

How long must one practice a perfect memory, a perfect imagination or study the latest manifestation of perfect sight?

The answer to this question is a benefit to the patient.

Teach Others

Many teachers have told me that when they taught Arithmetic the one who learned the most was always the teacher. Some ministers have made the remark that the one who profited mostly by the sermon was the man who delivered it.

For many years my patients who have been benefited by treatment without glasses have to a greater or less extent enjoyed the pleasure of helping others. When you think that you understand how to practice the swing with benefit try to teach somebody else how to do it. If you find palming is beneficial find how many of your friends who are also benefited by palming. But when you meet someone who is not benefited by what you tell them to do, you have at this time an opportunity of helping not only your friend but your own eyes as well.

It seems a simple matter for you to close your eyes, rest them for a half hour or so and find that your sight is improved by the rest. However, there are some people who are not benefited appreciably by closing their eyes and resting them. One cause of failure is the memory of imperfect sight.

Many patients failed to improve because with their eyes closed they think too much of their failure to see. Patients who have improved materially usually can demonstrate that the memory of perfect sight is restful, while the memory of imperfect sight is a strain. If you have a nearsighted friend who can read ordinary print without difficulty at the near point and without glasses, you can spend an hour or two of activity in showing your friend how to demonstrate while regarding fine print that it is impossible to try to concentrate on a point without sooner or later making the sight worse, that it is impossible to remember, imagine or see stationary letters, that it is impossible to maintain normal vision with the eyes kept continuously open without blinking.

VARIOUS TOPICS

Notes:

R

E L

A X I

N T O S

E E I N G

C E N T R A L

C L A R I T Y

S H I F T T B L I

N K A N D B R E A T H E

© 2010 VISIONS OF JOY. NATURAL VISION HABITS PRACTICE CHART.

Made in the USA
Middletown, DE
27 August 2019